D1130971

LINKING HEALTH AND MENTAL HEALTH

Volume 2, Sage Annual Reviews of Community Mental Health

EDITORIAL BOARD

Sage Annual Reviews of Community Mental Health

Co-Editors: **Richard H. Price**
Community Psychology Program
University of Michigan

John Monahan
School of Law
University of Virginia

C. Clifford Attkisson
Dept. of Psychiatry
Langley Porter Institute
University of California
San Francisco

Morton Bard
Center for Social Research
City University of New York

Bernard L. Bloom
Dept. of Psychology
University of Colorado

Stanley L. Brodsky
Dept. of Psychology
University of Alabama

Anthony Broskowski
Northside Community Mental
Health Center, Inc.
Tampa, Florida

Saul Cooper
Washtenaw County
Community Mental Health Center
Ann Arbor, Michigan

Emory L. Cowen
Dept. of Psychology
University of Rochester

Barbara Dohrenwend
Division of Sociomedical Sciences
School of Public Health
Columbia University

Kenneth Heller
Dept. of Psychology
Indiana University
Bloomington

Murray Levine
Dept. of Psychology
State University of New York
Buffalo

Ricardo F. Munoz
Social & Community Psychiatry Program
University of California, San Francisco &
San Francisco General Hospital

Amado M. Padilla
Dept. of Psychology
University of California
Los Angeles

Thomas F.A. Plaut
National Institute of Mental Health

N. Dickon Reppucci
Dept. of Psychology
University of Virginia

Stanley Sue
Dept. of Psychology
University of Washington

Carolyn F. Swift
National Council of Community
Mental Health Centers &
Southwest CMHC, Columbus, Ohio

Edison J. Trickett
Dept. of Psychology
University of Maryland

Volume 2
SAGE Annual Reviews of Community Mental Health

LINKING
HEALTH
and
MENTAL
HEALTH

edited by
Anthony Broskowski
Edward Marks
Simon H. Budman

MAR 18 1982

SAGE PUBLICATIONS   Beverly Hills   London

Copyright ©1981 by Sage Publications, Inc.

All rights reserved. No part of this book may be reproduced or utilized in any form or by any means, electronic or mechanical, including photocopying, recording, or by any information storage and retrieval system, without permission in writing from the publisher.

For information address:

SAGE Publications, Inc.
275 South Beverly Drive
Beverly Hills, California 90212

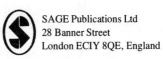

SAGE Publications Ltd
28 Banner Street
London ECIY 8QE, England

Printed in the United States of America

Library of Congress Cataloging in Publication Data

Library of Congress Cataloging in Publication Data
 Main entry under title:
 Linking health and mental health.

  (Sage annual reviews of community mental health; v. 2)
  Bibliography: p.
  1. Mental health services. 2. Medical cooperation. 3. Medical care. I. Broskowski, Anthony. II. Marks, Edward S. III. Budman, Simon. IV. Series. [DNLM: 1. Community health services. 2. Community mental health services. W1 SA125TC v. 2 / WM 30 L756]
  RA790.5.L57   362.2'068   81-8875
  ISBN 0-8039-1600-0   AACR2
  ISBN 0-8039-1601-9 (pbk.)

FIRST PRINTING

Contents

*To our parents —who understood
the mind-body connection*

Series Editors' Foreword

This second volume of *Sage Annual Reviews of Community Mental Health*, edited by Broskowski, Marks, and Budman, addresses a critical issue that will affect the future of the mental health system in the United States for some years to come. For several decades our health and mental health systems have operated on somewhat separate trajectories. This has been true despite the fact that a substantial proportion of mental health care has been delivered by primary medical care practitioners. In addition, many of the groups served by the mental health care system are not easily separated into those needing mental health and those needing generic health care services. All too often the results of the separation of mental health and health care have been inadequate care and fragmented services.

We are living in an age of soaring costs for health care and a corresponding concern for cost containment. At the same time, the pressure for more specialization among health and mental health care disciplines increases. Increased specialization can have an impact on attempts to understand the possible areas of common interest between the health and mental health fields. Whether the impact is positive or negative may depend less on specialized knowledge than on the recognition that our clients are people with a broad array of human and social needs.

In the past, the term "medical model" has been used as a kind of shorthand critique by many mental health professionals who believed that complex human problems were too often dismissed as "illnesses." Now, however, the mental health field appears to be going beyond this critique and asking serious and detailed questions about ways in which behavioral science can contribute to medical care as well as how medical care systems can improve the quality of lives of individuals in the community.

9

Broskowski and his colleagues have produced a book on the cutting edge of the field of health and mental health. The book amply documents the value of coordinating the health and mental health care systems, and suggests that coordination can have an impact on the quality of care and on the cost of that care. Professionals concerned with both health and mental health will find much of value in this volume. Because these issues cut across many disciplines, this volume should be valuable to social workers, nurses, psychiatrists, psychologists, health planners, and medical care administrators. It is a book which points the way to a better-integrated system of care and which recognizes the unique contributions of both mental health and health oriented professionals in enhancing the quality of life and health for each of us.

—Richard H. Price
John Monahan

PART I

INTRODUCTION AND OVERVIEW

1

The Health-Mental Health Connection

An Introduction

Anthony Broskowski
Northside Community Mental Health Center, Inc.
Tampa, Florida

This book is about the problems and prospects of coordinating health and mental health care. The coordination of these services will require coordination in related areas: planning, administration, training, and research. Most readers who have picked up this book are probably already open to considering this topic as a problem needing solutions. Others may want some persuasive arguments.

Each chapter, to some extent, sketches the dimensions of one or more problems associated with no coordination or poor coordination. At the level of the individual seeking help for poorly understood or self-diagnosed problems, a highly specialized or fragmented service system tends to reduce accessibility, accurate assessment, early intervention, treatment effectiveness, and on-going continuity of care. The most global index of societal benefit, the quality of our lives, must surely be diminished when health and mental health services are so organized as to reduce their effectiveness. Costs, of course, go up when inefficiencies occur and when ineffective outcomes must be repeatedly reassessed and redone. While knowledge in some delimited areas is advanced by specialization, a case will be made for the gains in knowledge realized by investigations that bridge separated specialties. Training and skill acquisition also tends to be organized in academic systems to achieve some initial, internal efficiencies at the expense of subsequent discontinuities and costs for service recipients—and professional rivalry and obsolesence.

If poor coordination produces problems, we would also argue that overintegration, or total consolidation, would create an equally negative state of affairs. This book is *not* about ignoring useful distinctions and eliminating all organizational separations of health and mental health resources. We may be visionary, but we are not revolutionists!

Forces Promoting Specialization

The mind-body distinction is an ancient and widely accepted dichotomy. It was strongly reinforced at the level of the federal government after World War II, when separate "institutes" for the various health specialties were created, including the National Institute for Mental Health. These actions were only a minor expression of a growing trend in this country to establish separate, categorical solutions for every significant problem coming to the attention of government administrators and legislators. Beginning in 1798, when the federal government established and operated the first merchant seaman hospital in Boston, the human service programs of the federal government slowly grew, undergoing numerous expansions, consolidations, and reorganizations (Attkisson & Broskowski, 1978). After World War II there was an accelerated rate of growth. By 1960 there were over 100 categorical programs in the Department of Health, Education and Welfare. By 1973 there were over 300 programs. Between 1965 and 1975 DHEW's share of the federal government's costs rose from less than 20 to 33 percent (Attkisson & Broskowski, 1978). In 1980 the Department of Education was elevated to Cabinet status and the Department of Health and Human Services (DHHS) was the new name for what was left. Will the future be any different?

This tendency toward growth and specialization, and its resultant fragmentation, inefficiency, and discontinuity, is also played out at levels of state and local government and in multiple institutions, universities, and service agencies. At last count in 1973, the average state government had between 80 and 100 separate human service administrative agencies, and the average community had from 400 to 500 direct service unts or agencies that were sponsored or funded by the government (Richardson, 1973).

These observations are not intended as an indictment of governmental concern for citizens but as a backdrop against which we can understand the general forces that promote and maintain the separation of the health and mental health sectors. We believe that the roots of the problem, if one will accept for the moment that it is a problem, can be traced to some generic, as well as specific, forces acting in systems and particularly in contemporary American society.

"Differentiation and specialization are common human responses for coping with complex and not very well understood phenomena" (Yessian & Broskowski, 1977: 271). The human body, and human feelings and behaviors, are extremely complex and poorly understood, not to mention highly valued. The search for reliable knowledge has promoted specialization, partly to ease and quicken the discovery process, partly to handle the storage and retrieval of facts as they accumulated. No one person is capable of maintaining depth and breadth in a world of exploding knowledge. Unfortunately, specialization in research tends to have two perhaps unintentional side effects. First, it promotes and reinforces specialization in the knowledge *application* process. For example, specialized research in health and illness tends to promote specialized delivery of health care services. Second, there is little conscious effort to ask research questions that cut across separate specialties. For example, how does the chemistry of the brain and cells affect behavior? When such cross-cutting questions begin to be asked, we invariably create a new specialized research and service application area to answer them. Specialization as a knowledge discovery strategy is not intrinsically wrong or damaging, provided we can balance that tendency with emphases, incentives, and strategies for integration, coordination, and generalization of findings into application.

"Generalists find it difficult to demonstrate the utility of their contributions" (Yessian & Broskowski, 1977: 272). The benefits of integration are seldom apparent in an immediate fashion. Rather, they are likely to be less dramatic, more subtle, take time, be difficult to evaluate, and be untraceable to any single individual. Patience is not valued in an environment of rapid change, and modesty seldom couples with ambition. New medical discoveries or new mental health interventions are likely to be well publicized, while directing a well-managed multiservice agency (perhaps an oxymoronic endeavor) is likely to go unnoticed. This second problem root is related to a third.

"Career rewards go to those who specialize" (Yessian & Broskowski, 1977: 273). Although profit-making industries pay their highest salaries to their "general managers," the human services sectors, governmental and private nonprofit, continue to give recognition and reward to their specialists. In some respects, specialization is easier. For career advancement it requires less effort to stay current, once an initial educational plateau is reached. Refining established research or treatment methods is less risky and hence more probable to lead to professional recognition and reward. One exception to this general rule is the rare person who achieves recognition by combining, integrating, or synthesizing two or more previously separated fields of endeavor, such as Jacob Bronowski, author of *The Ascent of Man* (1973). Major scientific and service advances have also come about in that fashion and are duly rewarded. However, a fundamental integration is a long shot on which few will risk their time and reputation.

"Legislators at the federal, state, and local levels are easily induced by the lure of categorical legislation" (Yessian & Broskowski, 1977: 273). Although this observation may be losing validity since it was written in 1977, it remains an accurate representation in most circumstances. Since 1960 the U.S. Congress enacted more than 400 categorical programs designed to meet specialized and narrowly defined needs of potential service recipients, professional providers, or researchers. The executive branch of government also tends to create specialized units, rules, and procedures in their search for a "quick fix." The scarcity of resources and the chaos of complexity are finally beginning to backwash the flow of narrow, categorical thinking in government. But special interest groups, some of which were spawned by earlier legislation, will continue to lobby mightily to maintain their unique and specialized existences and their care and feeding by government. Schon (1971) vividly describes just such assertive action to remain the same as "dynamic conservatism." Unfortunately, "dynamic conservatism" also leads to active aggression as resources dwindle. One profession must begin to fight another to increase or maintain its share.

Emanating from growing concerns with service fragmentation, inaccessibility, discontinuity, duplication, and inefficiency, major efforts were made in the 1960s and 1970s at all levels of federal, state, and local government to better coordinate and integrate the entire range of human services being provided at the state and local levels. Some of the major efforts in this area, called Services Integration Projects, were funded by the Department of Health, Education and Welfare (Spencer, 1974). These efforts were characterized by large-scale plans to create integrated structures for policy-making, planning, funding, and service delivery. Most of these large-scale projects were subject to review and evaluation (John, 1977; Henton, 1979).

These general concerns for improved services coordination achieved greater focus with respect to special high-risk target groups and those persons who were likely to have greater than usual problems gaining access and continuity of care across specialized settings. Some of these specific concerns were then brought together by the President's Commission on Mental Health (1978). The commission's final report and associated appendices documented the continuing needs of high-risk groups which remained unserved or underserved. The reasons for these problems included the barriers to care presented by existing organizational service methods, the poor match between the distribution of needs and resources (facilities, programs, and service staff), and the continuing stigma associated with mental illness and the utilization of mental health services. The need to develop coordinated primary health and mental health delivery strategies was recognized particularly for such special high-risk groups as chronic psychiatric patients, children, migrants, the elderly, and other groups in which multiple needs and stigma are most predominant. Unfortunately, as illustrated by Hagedorn in Chapter 3, although integrated planning is commonly seen as a way of correcting the excesses of categorical programming, it fails to do so because of the emphasis placed on the participative and coordinated *processes* of planning rather than substantive changes in the delivery system.

The Rationale for Coordination

Several arguments can be made to support the importance of improving the coordination of health and mental health services. These arguments are arbitrarily organized by considering issues of service utilization, epidemiology, diagnostic and treatment practices, financial and organizational patterns, professional training, and research. Each is inextricably bound to the other.

Utilization and Epidemiology

The current realities of health and mental health service utilization patterns provide a cogent argument for planned changes in the system of fragmented service organization. There is evidence that, in fact, the greatest amount of mental health care is already being provided by the primary health care sector. Regier, Goldberg, and Taube (1978) estimate that approximately 54 percent of all persons seen for a diagnosed mental health disorder are seen exclusively in the primary care sector. Only 15 percent of all those persons with diagnosed mental health disorders (3 percent of the total population) receive services in the specialty mental health sector (e.g., CMHCs and psychiatric hospitals). Furthermore, a significant percentage of the primary care physican's caseload consists of patients with significant mental health problems as their chief or secondary complaint, and there is a positive correlation between the utilization of medical services and the presence of psychiatric problems. The extensive degree of overlap in the epidemiological and clinical domains of health and mental health are documented by Goplerud in Chapter 4.

An excellent review of the literature on the relationship of health and mental health disorders by Hankin and Oktay (1979) also documents the prevalence of mental disorders seen in primary care settings. Their literature review examines evidence for different hypotheses to account for the relatively high rate of medical service utilization by persons with psychiatric problems.

One hypothesis is that psychologically disturbed persons may have a lower tolerance of physical illness symptoms or greater "propensities to seek medical care" (Hankin & Oktay, 1979). Also, they may be more likely to somaticize their psychological problems. Some may actually incur more health problems than less psychologically disturbed, "normal" persons. For reasons not well understood, emotional difficulties could increase susceptibility to germs or make one more accident-prone (Broskowski & Baker, 1974).

Patients with emotional problems probably perceive less of a stigma when they seek care in a primary health care setting than when they encounter a mental health setting (Hankin and Oktay, 1979). Negative labeling and stigmatization are avoided by avoiding the mental health sector.

Finally, the findings that persons with emotional problems tend to use medical services at a higher than average rate can be partly explained by economic incentives. A visit to an internist for back pain and "tension" is more likely to be reimbursed, depending on the diagnosis and treatment reported to the insurance company, than would a visit to a community mental health center.

Diagnostic and Treatment Practices

Depending upon the personal interests, training, and diagnostic skills of the provider, or the organizational setting, a single symptom or "problem" is likely to be isolated from all others, and only specialized services for that narrowly defined problem will be provided. Psychiatric disorders are commonly underdetected in health settings, and medical illnesses go undiagnosed in psychiatric settings, although a problem in either domain could be creating the symptoms of the other domain. A medical disease can be masked as a psychological disturbance, and psychological distress can "cause" or exacerbate somatic symptoms. Looking at such issues from a research perspective, Walker reviews the need for better knowledge to handle behavioral emergencies in Chapter 15.

Literature on the management of emotionally disturbed patients in primary care settings has also been reviewed by Hankin in an excellent edited volume of readings entitled *Mental Health Services in Primary Care Settings: Report of a Conference, April 2-3, 1979* (Parron & Solomon, 1980).

Her review indicates that there is a heavy reliance on the use of psychotropic medication by primary care physicians and that they commonly provide some brief psychotherapy, variously defined, to patients with emotional problems. Furthermore, the medical treatment regimen prescribed may or may not be followed depending upon psychological or behavior characteristics of the patient or the provider. Hankin reports that there is very little in the way of well-conducted research on the intensity, appropriateness, and effectiveness of these patient management techniques. The National Ambulatory Medical Care Survey shows that the nonpsychiatric physician spends an average of 13 minutes on each patient's visit (Hankin & Oktay, 1979). Clearly, the pace and volume of medical services in primary care settings preclude the intensity of mental health diagnosis and treatment methods found in typical, specialty mental health settings.

Finally, there is a growing literature on behavioral medicine and those environmental and behavioral factors that are related to general levels of health or specific diseases. Stress, diet, exercise, smoking, and a host of psychological factors are being implicated in an increasingly greater range of medical disorders previously thought to be related exclusively to genetic, biological, or chemical factors (Houpt, Orleans, George, & Brodie, 1979; Stone, Cohen, & Adler, 1979). Greater awareness of the role of psychological and behavioral factors in general health and medical care will continue to suggest a greater cooperation between specialty mental health professionals and both general and specialty medical professionals. Clearly, we are likely to witness increasing use of behavioral interventions, such as exercise, meditation, and changes in lifestyles and habits, as adjuncts or substitutes for orthodox medical treatment, such as drugs and surgery. Psychologically based interventions will also be used to improve patient compliance, speed recovery from necessary but disruptive medical procedures (e.g., surgery), or manage patients with chronic or terminal disease processes. Psychological interventions will be used for illness *prevention* or health enhancement. For an excellent example of such activities, we recommend Chapter 8 by James Manuso.

Financing Services

In addition to the current realities of epidemiology, utilization, and professional practice patterns, there is continuing pressure to reexamine and change existing methods of service organization and financing. Health Maintenance Organizations (HMOs), health care foundations, health/mental health group practices, and new cost containment and financial incentive systems are receiving great attention. The heavy utilization of medical services by persons with psychiatric problems suggests that significant cost savings may be realized when less expensive and more appropriate mental health services are made available as an alternative to expensive and unnecessary medical services. Extensive literature and research related to these issues have been discussed under the rubric of "cost offset." While there is evidence that medical care utilization is reduced following mental health interventions, major logical and methodological barriers must be surmounted before we can arrive at a reliable estimate of the size of the offset effect and achieve a valid understanding of its causes. For example, is there a selective reduction of only *inappropriate* medical utilization, and do patients receiving mental health interventions maintain adequate health levels without medical interventions? Many of these difficulties are spelled out by Mumford, Schlesinger, and Glass in Chapter 14.

Service utilization and cost patterns are also motivating a shift away from long-term institutionally based care toward short-term, ambulatory—or home-based—community care. Priorities for exotic and costly acute medical diagnostic equipment and treatment regimens are being increasingly challenged. Health education approaches, self-care, and prevention will undoubtedly receive more attention, even if only for the sake of the political rhetoric and rationale needed to cut government subsidies of health care. Dramatic alternatives to promote effectiveness and cost containment are suggested by Yates and DeMuth in Chapter 5.

Organization of Services

The National Health Planning and Resource Development Act of 1974 mandated that the Department of Health, Education and Welfare (now DHHS) develop national health planning goals. These were finally published in the November 25, 1980 issue of *The Federal Register*. Besides calling for continued cost-control planning procedures throughout the entire health service spectrum, these goals specifically identify mental health concerns and recommend "in-service mental health training of primary care providers and placement of mental health professionals in primary care programs." The goals call for the organization of mental health, drug abuse, and alcoholism services that will improve their coordination with the mainstream of health care.

This federal document is just one of many appearing on the scene each day that recommend closer ties between primary health care and mental health care. Obviously, these recommendations imply closer organizational and professional cooperation. Chapter 2, by Burns, Burke, and Kessler, spells out additional federal government efforts to promote coordination.

Organizational approaches toward coordination can vary considerably, depending on local resources and interests. Research conducted in the earliest days of the Community Health Centers Program demonstrated that the most consistent barrier to the goal of achieving comprehensive neighborhood health services was the lack of mental health services (Langston, 1979). This study further concluded that the lack of available personnel and the general stigma of mental health contribute to the gaps between need, demand, and actual utilization.

During the 1960s and 1970s many models were designed and tested to overcome service fragmentation or duplication of effort. Centralized information and referral systems, centralized diagnostic and evaluation services, the one-stop, multiservice center, and single case managers and advocates were among the popular experiments in broad-based coordinated care during the seventies. More modest attempts, however, have generally been more successful (Broskowski, 1980). *Intra*organizational team models, or written *inter*organizational agreements between a few health and mental health agencies to exchange specific resources (i.e., clients, staff, space, money, support services, transportation, equipment), are a recommended place to begin making the necessary institutional changes.

There are many mechanisms available to achieve varying levels of coordination. A few examples are multidisciplinary teams within an organization, liaison staff between two or more separate units within an organization or between separate organizations (e.g., a neighborhood health center and a community mental health center); integrated clinical records; case- or program-centered consultation services; joint intake, assessment, and triage functions; and collaborative treatment or case-management services. If liaison or consultation staff are used, these professionals must be adequately trained to develop and maintain good relationships across disciplinary boundaries and have the necessary clinical skills, patience, and tolerance for differences that will win respect on both sides of the linkage (Broskowski, 1980). In Chapter 6 Budman describes alternative models of providing mental health services in an HMO. Wertlieb, in Chapter 7, describes a range of services to be provided by mental health specialists in primary care settings. Innovative organizational arrangements and service programs within a private insurance company are described by Manuso in Chapter 8.

Most *inter*organizational agreements will hinge on both *administrative* concerns, such as the exchange of money for services, and *clinical* concerns, such as which professional of which organization will maintain clinical authority and supervisory control. Such agreements must be arrived at by a firm but incremental process. Differences in their respective service methods, vocabularies, and treatment ideologies can present formidable, but undiscussed, barriers to cooperative ventures among health and mental health staff. Allegiance to a common model, such as an integrated biopsychosocial model, does help enormously where and whenever it can be achieved. Greater detail on these and other organizational issues are presented in Chapter 9 by Marks and Broskowski.

Continuing barriers to coordinate health and mental health care are the interdisciplinary rivalries within the mental health sector or within the health sector. For example, family medicine is experiencing a renewed priority at the national level but may have to compete vigorously at the local level with organized medicine, medical schools, hospitals, or other medical specialties (such as surgery) for a larger share of resources, (space, equipment, students, faculty slots, curriculum content, etc.). Tensions within the medical profession grow as fewer medical students choose psychiatry as a specialty and psychiatry departments are threatened with a diminishing quantity and quality of residents. Simultaneously, mental health professionals fight one another over licensing and reimbursement issues. How much these struggles may hinder coordinated care is illustrated by the attempts to prevent psychologists from having hospital-admitting or consultation privileges. This lack of professional stature for professional psychologists can, in turn, reduce their ability to collaborate effectively with physicians whose patients are being hospitalized. Also, if psychiatry's status is being threatened by family medicine, this is likely to stimulate efforts by organized psychiatry to limit or control competition from other mental health disciplines which have effective and inexpensive contributions to make toward coordinated care. The real tragedy in all of these struggles is the energy that is wasted by interdisciplinary warfare that could be directed toward cooperative solutions and strategies for coordinated care.

Training Concerns

Moving upstream from the point where professionals, both clinicians and administrators, must work together as agency employees or private practitioners, concerns shift to the need to coordinate professional didactic and field-based training experiences. Social and behavioral science courses are now commonly required in medical student education. Family medicine and other primary care fields are beginning to include training on the diagnosis and treatment of mental health problems. Nurse practitioners, physician assistants, and a host of ancillary medical personnel are being trained with a greater awareness of social, behavioral, and emotional correlates of medical illness (Brown & Regier, 1977). Psychiatry's historical links to medicine are being rediscovered, and medical-psychiatric liaison work is receiving renewed attention.

Psychology and social work training programs are beginning to include more material on health, health care, and health policy and planning. In some cases, specialized tracks in medical social work or health psychology are being implemented (Stone et al., 1979). More field-based training, at both the pre- and postgraduate level, and continuing professional education must be based on conjoint professional training and supervision. Chapter 10 by Hollen, Ehrlich, and White, Chapter 11 by Authier, and Chapter 12 by Stone address these training concerns.

Research Issues

Considerable research needs to be done on the health-mental health connection. Thus, research is needed on the *epidemiology* of health/mental health. What is the estimated incidence and prevalence of conjoint health/ mental health problems? How do such estimates vary with different measurement methods, research designs, or service settings? Do some problems more commonly co-occur than others? Do certain psychological or environmental conditions (e.g., high rates of change, noise, stress) have a predictable outcome with respect to medical conditions? What are the early developmental conditions associated with poor health and health behaviors in later adult life?

Treatment research can examine the effectiveness of alternative psychological and behavioral interventions on various disease processes or specific syndromes. Alternative *patient management* strategies can be compared with one another. For example, what are the relative costs and rates of effectiveness of family medicine physicians providing brief psychotherapy for depressed patients compared with a procedure emphasizing drug therapy and referral to a mental health specialist?

Alternative *organizational* and *financial* arrangements deserve systematic evaluation for their relative contributions to accessibility, continuity, and effectiveness of care. What are the costs and effects of financial incentives for organizations and their professional staff to provide coordinated care? Will citizens make better judgments about the relative contribution of biological and psychological factors to their health and well-being, and make better choices for treatment, if they are provided with education and financial incentives to seek optimal care? Will organized health promotion strategies emphasizing lifestyle changes, including changes in physical environment, behavior, and social relations, improve statistics on morbidity and mortality? What evidence will Congress demand before reallocating its fiscal priorities from dramatic, acute conditions (e.g., cancer) toward coordinated care of more prevalent and costly chronic conditions, including mental illness and conditions associated with the aging process? Would coordinated care approaches have their greatest impact when focused on pathological conditions of infancy and childhood?

These are just a few examples of the many clinical, financial, and organizational jungles that need clearing and illumination through research; research that will require scientists and settings to be receptive to the challenge. Such issues are discussed in greater depth in Chapter 13 by Attkisson and Broskowski.

In summary, there is a wide spectrum of concerns about coordinated care: social policy and planning; clinical epidemiology and service utilization; organizational and financial mechanisms; and professional practice, training, and research. The field is just beginning to be explored, and the potential risks and benefits are enormous! If the reader is excited about learning something new, a challenge that goes beyond specialization, then we encourage you to read further.

References

Attkisson, D. C., & Broskowski, A. Evaluation and the emerging human service concept. In C. C. Attkisson, W. Hargreaves, M. Horowitz, & J. Sorenson (Eds.), *Evaluation of human service programs*. New York: Academic Press, 1978.

Bronowski, J. *The ascent of man*. Boston: Little, Brown, 1973.

Brown, B., & Regier, D. How NIMH now views the primary care physician. *Practical Psychology for Physicians*, 1977, 5, 12-14.

Broskowski, A. Literature review on interorganizational relationships and their relevance to health and mental health coordination. Final contract report to NIMH, Contract No. 278-79-0030(OP). Rockville, Maryland, 1980.

Broskowski, A., & Baker, F. Professional, organizational, and social barriers to primary prevention. *American Journal of Orthopsychiatry*, 1974, 44, 707-719.

Hankin, J., & Oktay, J. S. *Mental disorder and primary medical care: An analytic review of the literature*. National Institute of Mental Health, Series D, No. 5, DHEW Pub. No. (ADM) 78-661. Washington, DC: Government Printing Office, 1979.

Henton, D. *The feasibility of services integration*. Berkeley: University of California Press, 1975.

Houpt, J., Orleans, C., George, L., & Brodie, K. *The importance of mental health services to general health care*. Cambridge, MA: Ballinger, 1979.

John, D. *Managing the human service system: What have we learned from services integration?* Project SHARE Monograph Series, No. 4. Rockville, Maryland, 1977.

Langston, J.H. The neighborhood health center program. In J.G. Abert (Ed.), *Program evaluation at HEW: Research versus reality. Part 1: Health.* New York: Marcel Dekker, Inc., 1979.

Parron, D.L., & Solomon, F. (Eds.). *Mental health services in primary care settings: Report of a conference, April 2-3, 1979, Washington, D.C.* National Institute of Mental Health, Series DN, No. 2, DHHS Publication No. (ADM) 80-995. Washington, DC: Government Printing Office, 1980.

President's Commission on Mental Health. Report to the President. Washington, DC: Government Printing Office, 1978.

Regier, D.A., Goldberg, I.D., & Taube, C.A. The de facto U.S. mental health services system. *Archives of General Psychiatry,* 1978, 35, 685-693.

Richardson, E.R. Responsibility and responsiveness (II): A report on the HEW potential for the seventies. Memorandum of the Secretary of Health, Education and Welfare, January 19. Washington, DC: DHEW, 1973.

Schon, D.A. *Beyond the stable state.* New York: W.W. Norton, 1971.

Spencer, L., Jr. The federal approach to services integration. *Urban Social and Change Review,* 1974, 7, 7-13.

Stone, G., Cohen, R., & Adler, N. *Health psychology–A handbook.* San Francisco: Jossey-Bass, 1979.

Yessian M., & Broskowski, A. Generalists in human-service systems: Their problems and prospects. *Social Science Review,* 1977, 51, 265-288.

2

Promoting Health-Mental Health Coordination

Federal Efforts

Barbara J. Burns
Jack D. Burke, Jr.
Larry G. Kessler
Primary Care Research Section
National Institute of Mental Health

In the past decade federal policies have demonstrated increased recognition of the benefits to be gained from coordinating health and mental health care. As evidence has grown about the effectiveness of coordinated health and mental health care, both legislative and administrative bodies have expanded efforts to promote coordinated care. These initiatives have dealt with service delivery, training for future service delivery needs, and research on a wide range of related topics. Since the initial positive assessment of the different programs suggests that these efforts will be strengthened in the future, especially after implementation of the Mental Health Systems Act of 1980 (PL 96-398), we plan to discuss recent federal initiatives to promote coordinated care through service delivery systems, support of training efforts, and additional research. Our discussion will focus mainly on programs related to the National Institute of Mental Health.

The Need for Coordinated
General Health-Mental Health Care

The rationale for these policies has developed from a convergence of three different lines of argument (Burke, Burns, O'Flaherty, & Broskowski,

---

AUTHOR'S NOTE: This chapter is in the public domain and may be reproduced without the permission of the authors or the publisher.

1980). First, within medicine generally, the interrelationship between medical and psychological problems has won wider acknowledgment (Eisenberg, 1979). This relationship has been discussed from several perspectives: Physical and psychological problems can coexist in the same patient; physical problems can produce secondary emotional reactions; psychological and behavioral problems can lead directly to poor physical health; and both physical and psychiatric conditions can serve as hidden causes or as complications of each other (Houpt, Orleans, George, & Brodie, 1979; Shepherd, 1980). Although these associations are recognized, recent studies have provided increased evidence of the importance of co-occuring mental and physical disorders (Vaillant, 1979; Andrews, Schonell, & Tennant, 1977) in general medical populations.

Second, from the perspective of studies done on patient use of general health services, a close relationship between mental and physical disorders has been further highlighted. In the United States, it has been estimated that at least 15 percent of all patients seen by primary care physicians have diagnosable mental disorders and that 60 percent of all patients in the United States with emotional problems are seen in the general health/primary care sector. Of this group of patients, only 10 percent receive additional services in the mental health specialty sector, so 54 percent of patients in this country with emotional problems are seen exclusively by primary care clinicians (Regier, Goldberg, & Taube, 1978).

Third, from the perspective of research studies assessing effectiveness of coordinated care, several areas of investigation suggest that actually providing integrated general health-mental health services leads to more effective patient care. In a study of a comprehensive neighborhood health center in Boston, where integrated general and mental health care was provided, it was shown that community residents were much more likely to receive outpatient mental health care than in surveys of outpatient mental health services generally (Jacobson, Regier, & Burns, 1978). In a direct effort to measure patient outcome, investigators in Great Britain demonstrated that providing psychiatric and social work services in a general practice led to improved clinical and social functioning among patients having a "chronic neurosis," as compared with control patients (Cooper, Harwin, Depla, & Shepherd, 1975).

Federal Policies to Promote
Coordination of Care

In its report to the President, the President's Commission on Mental Health proposed comprehensive and far-reaching recommendations for the development of mental health services throughout the nation. One of its conclusions was that "greater attention must be paid to the relationship between health and mental health" (President's Commission, 1978: 20), and the commission recommended the establishment of "cooperative working arrangements between health care settings and community mental health service programs" to further that aim. Besides recommending increased training of mental health personnel, the commission recommended increased funding for mental health training of "primary health care givers and students" (1978: 39). To enhance understanding of how mental health services are currently provided and how they should be provided in the future, it also recommended expanded research on mental health service delivery systems (1978: 49).

Partly as a response to the commission's report to the President, the National Institute of Mental Health (NIMH) and the Bureau of Community Health Services (BCHS) joined in April 1979 with the Institute of Medicine to sponsor a two-day international conference, on issues related to coordinating health and mental health care (Parron & Solomon, 1980; Borus, Burns, Jacobson, Macht, Morrill, & Wilson, 1980). One of the working papers at that conference, which had been prepared as a background paper for the President's Commission on Mental Health, described the experiences of 19 neighborhood health centers in Boston which had joint general health services. In that paper, Borus and colleagues described the wide range of benefits to be gained in integrated care and the range of approaches to coordinating care which can be taken between general health and mental health facilities. They summarized the benefits of general health-mental health coordination as improved case finding, more successful referrals, increased integration of care, and better follow-up of patients (Borus et al., 1980).

To make these benefits more widely available, a series of administrative and legislative programs have been designed to encourage greater coordination of general health and mental health care. The Carter Administration sponsored, besides several administrative initiatives, the Mental Health Systems Act of 1980 to implement the major proposals of the President's Commission on Mental Health. Significantly, one of the priorities of this act is to increase the provision of mental health services in health care centers, beginning in fiscal 1982.

Service Delivery

In the past 15 years, the federal government has developed and supported two parallel systems of ambulatory health care centers—for general health care and for mental health care. During the 1960s, to provide general health care, legislation for the Office of Economic Opportunity established primary care health centers, such as neighborhood health centers and family health centers. In 1967, Section 314 of the Public Health Service Act established health centers known as "Primary Care Centers." In 1975, PL 94-63 added Section 330 to the Public Health Service Act to sponsor primary health care centers in medically underserved areas. Today, in terms of general health care, the Bureau of Community Health Services sponsors about 1000 primary health care projects (PHCPs) in medically underserved urban and rural areas of the country. To provide mental health care, the first community mental health centers (CMHCs) were created in 1963 after President Kennedy sponsored the Community Mental Health Act in 1962. In 1975, PL 94-63 also added amendments to the act and expanded the scope of activities. Today, in terms of outpatient mental health services, the National Institute of Mental Health sponsors 744 community mental health centers which are intended to serve all residents within a geographically defined catchment area.

Although the legislation for both general health and mental health centers implies the need for coordination of services and comprehensive care, funding specifically targeted toward facilitating coordinated care between centers was not available until very recently. Several factors made coordination difficult. Besides being sponsored by different federal agencies and receiving different kinds of funding, these two types of centers serve populations defined in different ways. The primary health care projects serve populations defined according to target characteristics, such as the rural poor; CMHCs, however, serve much larger population bases, of about 75,000-200,000 people, including everyone living within the catchment area. To overcome the tendency of PHCPs and CMHCs to operate in isolation from each other, BCHS and NIMH began a linkage initiative in fiscal 1978 to enable the PHCPs to hire mental health specialists to serve as liaison "linkage workers" with the local CMHC. Initially, 50 PHCPs received grants of as much as $30,000 to hire a mental health linkage worker. By spring 1980, 47 of these centers had linkage programs still operating, and in fiscal 1980 an additional 65 grants were made to new centers to hire linkage workers. In fiscal 1981, both BCHS and NIMH plan to contribute funding to expand the linkage program to a new group of centers.

Initial program experience has demonstrated that the local projects receiving grants have implemented the linkage program in different ways. For example, in rural areas where the health center is located at some distance from the local CMHC, a linkage worker might be expected to provide consultation to primary care clinicians and to provide counseling and brief therapy to patients with emotional problems. In large, urban PHCPs, linkage workers often tend to concentrate on developing good referral mechanisms to the local CMHC and on providing evaluation, referral, and follow-up services for patients from the PHCP.

Preliminary results from a descriptive survey of these 47 programs (Broskowski, 1980; Goldman, Burns, & Burke, 1980) in spring 1980 reveal that center administrators believe the linkage initiative has had many of the desired effects, such as increasing primary care clinicians' awareness and detection of emotional problems, increasing the proportion of health center patients who receive mental health services, and producing more appropriate use of health and mental health services. However, definitive assessment of these changes must await more rigorous studies.

At the same time, several kinds of problems have been reported by center administrators and linkage workers, and these problems indicate areas where assistance and guidance can be provided to linkage grant recipients. Agreeing on objectives of the program, and arranging to share administrative responsibility for it, were cited as frequent early problems. These problems might have been exacerbated by the potential in the grant program to concentrate the resources (i.e., funds and linkage worker services) in the health center exclusively while also producing increased patient referrals to the CMHC. In half the cases, this potential problem was apparently resolved by assuring joint supervision of the linkage worker by the two centers, by having the linkage worker provide some direct patient services at the health center without referring all patients to the CMHC, and by having the linkage worker provide some services to patients at the CMHC.

Other problems cited, especially in rural areas, were practical difficulties in arranging patient transportation between the two centers, sharing medical record information, and providing private office space to the linkage worker. In some of these rural programs, a difficult problem was recruiting qualified linkage workers. More than half of the linkage workers were relatively inexperienced, with less than five years of clinical experience in mental health. Adjusting to a "foreign" setting like an ambulatory health center was a trying experience for many of them (Burke et al., 1980; for further details, see Chapter 9 of this volume).

In response to these problems, the National Institute of Mental Health has planned a national technical assistance resource center on linkages to provide guidance and information both to federally sponsored linkage programs and to other facilities such as county health departments, nursing homes, and other health care facilities which can benefit from coordinating health and mental health care.

As a result of the apparent success of this linkage initiative, and in anticipation of the Mental Health Systems Act, the administrators of the Alcohol, Drug Abuse, and Mental Health Administration and of the Health Services Administration (which are the parent agencies of NIMH and BCHS, respectively) signed an agreement on June 23, 1980, pledging their agencies to expand linkage activities in a broad range of service and training areas. This agreement also established an ADAMHA-HSA coordinating committee to meet regularly, share information, explore new initiatives, and monitor the progress of existing programs. Among the various projects included in the agreement are efforts to enlarge the NIMH-BCHS Linkage Initiative (including expansion to include alcohol and drug abuse services); to expand linkages to include CMHCs and Public Health Service (PHS) outpatient clinics at PHS hospitals supported by the Bureau of Medical Services; and to sponsor joint programs to train primary care providers in HSA clinics to increase their awareness and understanding of alcohol, drug abuse, and mental health problems (HSA-ADAMHA, 1980).

As mentioned earlier, Section 206 of the Mental Health Systems Act of 1980 provides an authorization of $15 million to fund mental health services in health care centers in fiscal 1982, with even larger amounts in later years. With a much broader scope than the BCHS-NIMH Linkage Initiative, the Systems Act allows the Secretary of Health and Human Services to award such grants either to mental health centers or to health centers. These do not need to be federally supported centers, but can be any public or nonprofit entity providing either basic mental health services, as specified in the act, or a wide range of health services. In fact, such diverse health providers as hospital outpatient departments, skilled nursing homes, and health maintenance organizations are named as being among those eligible. This section of the act also allows other mental health professionals besides a linkage worker to be supported by the grant. With this increased flexibility in terms of centers eligible to apply and staff eligible for support, local centers will be able to structure general health/mental health programs closely suited to their own needs.

Training

Just as federal agencies have attempted to promote the delivery of coordinated care by health and mental health centers, a parallel federal effort has emphasized mental health training for primary care clinicians (PCC). Since primary care clinicians provide first-contact and continuing care, they have an unmatched opportunity to detect emotional problems early, to intervene promptly, and to arrange effective consultation-referral relationships with mental health specialists. For PCCs to fill this potential role, training throughout their careers must provide the necessary knowledge, attitudes, and skills for managing emotional problems through direct patient service and through continuing interaction with mental health specialists. Although the boundaries around this mental health role of PCCs have not yet been clearly drawn, either by research findings or by setting professional standards, the need for PCCs to respond to their patients' emotional problems has been well documented (Regier & Rosenfeld, 1977). This clear need has stimulated the development of legislation, administrative policy, and funding programs aimed at improving mental health training of PCCs.

The Health Professions Educational Assistance Act of 1976 stimulated policy and programs related to mental health training for PCCs. This act supported increased training of primary health care physicians (general internal medicine, family medicine, and general pediatrics), in contrast to medical specialists, and it also provided a number of training options in the general health-mental health area. These options included "the use of a team approach in the delivery of health services"; "establishing humanity in health care centers"; "cooperative human behavior and psychiatry in medical and dental education and practice"; "social work in health care"; "psychology training programs"; and "training in the diagnosis, treatment and prevention of diseases and related medical and behavioral problems of the aged." The act also encouraged mental health training in family practice residency programs and inclusion of psychiatry in area health education centers. As of October 1980, this act has technically expired, and widely differing versions of the bill have been under discussion in the House and Senate.

In 1976, in response to this legislation and to its own earlier interest in establishing new directions for its training programs, NIMH convened the Workgroup on Primary Care Training (Regier & Rosenfeld, 1977). Recommendations from the workgroup were incorporated into the ADAMHA Forward Plan, FY 1978-1982. The two fundamental recommendations were to expand mental health teaching in primary care residencies (including new support for mental health clinicians to do the teaching) and to support state manpower development programs which provide mental health training for practicing PCCs through continuing education.

These legislative and administrative initiatives have led to specific developments at three levels: within NIMH; between ADAMHA and HSA; and at the departmental level in the Department of Health and Human Services. Each of these efforts is described briefly.

At the NIMH level, the Mental Health Service Manpower Development and Training Grants announcements establish, as one of three basic priorities, "the development of mental health skills and knowledge of general health care personnel and preparing mental health specialists to work more effectively with the health care field" (NIMH, 1979b). These broad objectives for primary care are spelled out in relation to three types of grants: those applicable to the mental health disciplines; research and demonstration grants; and the manpower systems development grants, which support projects to provide continuing education for "primary care personnel to improve their capability to provide preventive, diagnostic, therapeutic, rehabilitative and supportive mental health services" (NIMH, 1979a).

NIMH has provided financial support related to the primary care focus for the four core mental health disciplines and paraprofessionals. The following data represent 1980 activities. The Psychiatry Education Branch, Division of Mental Health Training Programs, awarded $10.2 million in grants, or 48 percent of its budget, for programs related to the interface with general health; of this total, $5.1 million went for medical student education, $4.9 million for General Practice Special or Consultation/Liaison Programs, and $0.2 million for "other" primary care programs. The Psychology Education Branch spent $873,000 on psychology and general health training and reported an increase in the number of psychologist graduates (from NIMH-supported training programs) who have accepted positions in hospitals and medical schools. Eight social work projects with a primary health focus were funded by the Social Work Education Branch at a total cost of $570,000. One training center, for example, places social work students in medical group practices in the rural Ozarks of Missouri. The Nursing Branch funded 17 applications with a major primary care component at a cost of $683,000; of these, ten were for master's level programs, six for continuing education, and one for an undergraduate project. Paraprofessional training grants are supporting the mental health component of programs for physician assistants and emergency medical technicians in the states of Colorado, New York, and Nebraska for a total cost of $266,000 in 1980.

At the agency level, and closely tied to the aims of the NIMH Manpower Systems Development program, is the HSA-ADAMHA Memorandum of Understanding of June 23, 1980. The training aspect of this interagency agreement seeks to "strengthen the ability of the general health care sector to recognize, diagnose, and treat ADM disorders" (HSA-ADAMHA, 1980). Pilot experience in ADM training of primary care practitioners from PHCPs occurred in 1979 through a contract supported by both agencies. During 1980, in support of the HSA-ADAMHA agreement, NIMH sponsored continuing education for PCCs in the states of Maine, Michigan, and West Virginia. Such efforts are expected to increase dramatically in subsequent years.

At the HHS level, a policy statement on primary care-mental health training can be found in the National Health Planning Goals issued by the department (Department of Health and Human Services, 1980). In addition to other health goals, the report states:

> The integration of mental health services in general health care delivery programs should be increased through in-service mental health training of primary care providers and placement of mental health professionals in primary care programs [p. 31].

In conclusion, legislative, policy, and program developments have converged at the federal level to strengthen the mental health training of primary care clinicians. The extent and effectiveness of these efforts will depend greatly on the level of resources allocated, the duration of such initiatives, and responses by professional groups at national and local levels. As these new training initiatives get under way, it will be important to assess, on a longitudinal basis, the impact of such training on clinical patient care. It will also be important to assess similar efforts initiated by other governmental (e.g., the Health Resources Administration) and nongovernmental agencies and groups (e.g., the Rockefeller Foundation).

Research

NIMH-sponsored research, either conducted by institute investigators or supported through institute funding, has examined a variety of issues related to the coordination of health and mental health care. Specific research questions can be classified into four broad areas important for understanding the relationship between general health care and mental health care.

(1) Size of the problem. Early studies have attempted to measure the prevalence of emotional problems in general medical populations.

(2) Use of services. A large number of studies in different types of settings have examined whether patients with emotional problems might show different patterns of using general medical services than do other patients.

(3) Clinical practice. Understanding how primary care clinicians recognize, diagnose, and manage patients with emotional problems is an active area of current investigation. Examining the type and effectiveness of the care provided represents the next logical research area in patient management studies.

(4) Coordination of services. Determining how mental health services can best relate to general medical services has gained importance as a result

of the recent policy initiatives designed to stimulate coordination of care.

In addition to these four areas of study, a parallel effort to examine the need for general health care by patients seen in the mental health services sector has received some attention.

The substantive and methodologic aspects within each of these research areas will be discussed. Following this, major research questions of particular interest will be highlighted.

Prevalence

A fundamental question in previous studies has been how to establish the rates of emotional problems in a population of primary care patients. As with studies from the United Kingdom (Shepherd, Cooper, Brown, & Kalton, 1966), studies sponsored by NIMH have shown a wide range of these rates, with from 7 to 22 percent of patients reported by primary care physicians as having emotional problems. Most of these investigations have used just a few practice settings as primary data sources (Hankin & Oktay, 1979). Data from the National Ambulatory Medical Care Survey (NAMCS; Delozier, 1975), a national survey of office-based physicians conducted by the National Center for Health Statistics, has demonstrated that 4.4 percent of office visits are associated with a diagnosed mental disorder (Regier & Goldberg, 1976).

It has become clear that a range of factors is responsible for producing such a wide variation in estimated prevalence rates. In addition to some true variability among the patient populations studied, an additional influence is variation in such physician characteristics as personality and attitude toward mental illness (Marks, Goldberg, & Hillier, 1979).

Another important factor which produces varying estimates of prevalence has been the use of different criteria to determine whether a patient has an emotional problem. For example, in a recent study at Marshfield Medical Foundation, Hoeper and his colleagues (1979) showed that 1.8 percent of patients have a diagnosed mental disorder as recorded routinely by the clinician. However, an independent review of these physicians' notes in the medical record revealed that as many as 5.1 percent of patients had been recognized as having a mental disorder even though a formal diagnosis was not recorded. To compare these estimates with the most rigorous criteria applied in a standardized way, a structured psychiatric interview (Schedule for Affective Disorders and Schizophrenia; Endicott & Spitzer, 1978) was used in the same study to provide a current psychiatric diagnosis. These diagnoses were based on the Research Diagnostic Criteria, which form the basis of the new DSM-III classification system. A surprisingly high figure was obtained; about 27 percent of patients received at least one diagnosis of a psychiatric disorder based on the SADS interview.

Use of Services

Three major topics have been examined concerning the use of general medical services by patients with mental disorders.

It has been documented in a variety of settings that individuals with diagnosed mental disorders have much higher rates of medical utilization than those individuals without mental disorders. In these studies, patients with mental disorders have rates of using general medical services that are sometimes as much as 100 percent greater than rates for other patients (Regier et al., 1980). Whether this higher rate of services use reflects a greater need for medical care and is therefore appropriate is not clear.

Early federal research in the utilization area also examined what is known as the "offset" effect—that is, the fact that patients who receive psychiatric care appear to have lower rates of using medical services after beginning this treatment than they did before seeing a mental health professional. Considerable offset effects were detected in early studies (Goldberg, Krantz, & Locke, 1970); however, those studies used no comparison groups and thus were inconclusive. A number of methodological problems, such as lack of comparison groups, has plagued studies of the offset effect (Jones & Vischi, 1979). More recent evidence from a carefully designed study with a matched comparison group shows that there seems to be no general offset effect but that certain special subgroups of patients receiving psychiatric treatment— in particular those who have a few visits for psychotherapy—do exhibit significant declines in subsequent medical use (Goldberg, Allen, Kessler, Carey, Locke, & Cook, in press; for more information on the offset effect and its interpretation, see Chapter 14).

A more specific focus for research has been on the use of and prescribing patterns of psychotropic medications in the United States. This research has raised a number of serious questions regarding the need for additional coordination of health and mental health care. As a class, psychotropic medications are some of the most prescribed drugs in this country, and much of the prescribing is being done by nonpsychiatric physicians (Parry, Balter, Mellinger, Cisin, & Mannheimer, 1973). In some cases, reports have decried the presumed "overmedication" of the public, especially in regard to the minor tranquilizers.

Recognition, Diagnosis, and Management

Within the broad category of the management of mental disorders, several research issues are important: the detection and diagnosis of those disorders; referral from health to mental health providers; and the treatment of patients recognized as having mental or emotional problems. These have been addressed by NIMH-sponsored preliminary studies, and plans have been made to expand such research efforts to look at these areas more closely.

As noted earlier in the section on reported prevalence, nonpsychiatric physicians show wide variation in their ability to detect and their willingness to record mental disorders in their patients (Marks et al., 1979). One research effort designed to improve detection and recognition of mental disorders was conducted by David Goldberg (1980) in South Carolina. This research demonstrated that training primary care residents to use better interviewing methods improved their recognition of emotional problems.

Efforts are underway to refine brief screening instruments to assist nonpsychiatric physicians in the detection of mental disorder using, for example, the General Health Questionnaire (GHQ; Goldberg, 1978). In addition, the GHQ is being used currently in a study related to the recognition, referral, and treatment of mental disorders in a primary care population. This study is examining whether providing the results of screening instruments like the GHQ to general physicians improves their detection and management of mental disorders. Further studies to examine how patients are managed by primary care clinicians are in the planning stages.

Coordination of Services

One multiple-site study has been conducted examining health and mental health utilization in organized health care settings (Regier, Goldberg, Kessler, & Burns, 1980). Each setting represented a different approach to integrating health and mental health care. Despite substantial differences in organizational structure, populations served, and facilities, the rates of mental disorder diagnosed in all populations are higher than in settings without integrated general health and mental health services. A substantial association between a diagnosis of mental disorder and relatively high use of health services was also evident in all four settings. These findings suggest that the integrated organization of health and mental health services may indeed increase reporting of mental and emotional problems, and that these organizational arrangements may promote mental health services use among populations presumably needing care.

As discussed in terms of the BCHS-NIMH Linkage Initiative, understanding ways to integrate health and mental health care is an important area for further program development. Future stages in the evolution of these health-mental health linkage programs will clarify how linkage serves as one approach to providing coordinated care. Further studies comparing totally integrated with minimally linked settings will also be needed, especially in conjunction with the research questions on management already discussed.

Research Issues

In terms of prevalence, a more comprehensive view of the reasons for variability in prevalence estimates is clearly needed. To the extent that variation in prevalence rates represents true differences between settings, it will be important to identify characteristics associated with these differences (e.g., differing socioeconomic patterns of patient populations). Also important will be efforts to clarify the types of problems presented, especially in terms of a spectrum from formal psychiatric disorders, to psychological and behavioral problems (including reaction to disease or to stress), to social problems that bring patients to a primary care clinician.

A number of questions remain in the utilization area that are important to answer in relation to coordination of care: Are the high rates of medical use by those individuals with mental disorder appropriate? Do patients seen in settings with integrated health and mental health care at the same site show different patterns of using medical services than those seen in nonintegrated settings? Do health and mental health care substitute for one another when one type of care is unavailable or inaccessible?

It should be clear that research on the patient management of mental disorders related to coordinated health and mental health care has just begun. Most of the major research questions in the area are left unanswered: Which disorders can appropriately be managed by nonpsychiatric physicians? When is referral more appropriate than obtaining consultation or liaison services? Can outcome be improved by coordinating patient care through teams comprised both of nonpsychiatric and psychiatric health care providers?

All of the studies highlight the need for more advanced methodology, especially for accurate and convenient diagnostic instruments to identify patients with emotional problems in primary care settings. In addition to refinement of case-finding instruments, the development of a variety of outcome measures is needed. Assessing changes in patients and relating these changes to the care provided will be critical in the extension of research that focuses on patient management practices and the effects of coordinated care. A clear definition of "integrated" services and measures of the degree of integration are also needed; these can be used in conjunction with studies examining patient management to assess the effects of organizational structure on clinical care.

In summary, recent research studies have broadened our knowledge of the amount and diversity of mental disorders seen in health care settings. This perspective has stimulated research to examine the degree of integrated care in a variety of settings and its effect on patients seen in these settings. Although a considerable number of research questions remain in all areas of endeavor described in this section, the mandates for increased research on the general health-mental health interface and for improvements in service delivery to patients seeking general health care are clear.

Conclusion

With increasing understanding about the need to provide mental health care that is coordinated with the growing primary care sector in the United States, federal efforts have aimed toward service, training, and research. The Health-Mental Health Linkage Initiative for federally supported centers has been dramatically expanded by the Mental Health Systems Act of 1980, which provides support for promoting health/mental health coordination in a wide variety of settings. Training grants to medical and graduate schools by NIMH have emphasized teaching mental health specialists to work in primary care settings and primary care clinicians to gain increased skill in diagnosing, treating, and referring patients with emotional problems. Research programs, such as the one sponsored by the Primary Care Research Section at NIMH, have examined the prevalence and detection of emotional problems in primary care patients and will expand to identify ways of managing these patients and to assess benefits and problems of greater coordination of services.

Many of these efforts have benefited from exchanging ideas with colleagues in other countries. The increasing interest in primary care in the United States reflects similar trends in other parts of the world; and the service, training, and research experiences of these countries have stimulated the work done in the United States. For example, a great deal of research in the United Kingdom has produced methodological advances as well as much of our early knowledge about the mental health role of general practitioners. Especially valuable have been projects conducted by the World Health Organization. In collaboration with NIMH, WHO has conducted a project to devise a new classification of psychological symptoms and social problems which can be used by primary care clinicians to supplement the existing classification of diseases. WHO has also sponsored the Extended Mental Health Care Project to train primary care workers to manage emotional problems in areas where physicians, and especially psychiatrists, are scarce.

With the increasing federal emphasis on coordinated care, and with continued enrichment through international collaboration, it is hoped that the importance of mental health problems in primary care will become clearer and that the efforts to improve service, training, and research will lead to better patient care and more appropriate use of medical services.

References

Andrews, G., Schonell, M., & Tennant, C. The relation between physical, psychological, and social morbidity in a suburban community. *American Journal of Epidemiology,* 1977, 105, 324-329.

Borus, J. F., Burns, B. J., Jacobson, A. M., Macht, L. B., Morrill, R. G., & Wilson, E. M. *Coordinated mental health care in neighborhood health centers.* DHHS Publication No. (ADM) 80-996. Washington, DC: Government Printing Office, 1980.

Broskowski, A. Final report, evaluation of the PHCP-CMHC Linkage Initiative. NIMH Contract 278-79-0030 (OP).

Burke, J. D., Burns, B. J., O'Flaherty, H., & Broskowski, A. Linkage relationships in the Federal Health-Mental Health Linkage Initiative: Clinical and organizational aspects. Paper presented at the annual meeting of the American Psychiatric Association, San Francisco, California, 1980.

Cooper, B., Harwin, B. G., Depla, C., & Shepherd, M. Mental health care in the community: An evaluative study. *Psychological Medicine,* 1975, 5, 372-380.

Delozier, J. E. *National Ambulatory Medical Care Survey, 1973 summary, United States, May 1973-April 1974.* DHEW Publication No. (HRA) 767-1772, October. (Vital and health statistics: Series 13, data from the National Health Survey, No. 21.) Washington, DC: Government Printing Office, 1975.

Department of Health and Human Services. *National health planning goals: The national guidelines for health planning.* Washington, DC: Health Resources Administration, Public Health Service, DHHS, 1980.

Eisenberg, L. Interfaces between medicine and psychiatry. *Comprehensive Psychiatry,* 1979, 20, 1-14.

Endicott, J., & Spitzer, R. L. A diagnostic interview: The schedule for affective disorders and schizophrenia. *Archives of General Psychiatry,* 1978, 35, 837-844.

Goldberg, D. Manual of the General Health Questionnaire. Windsor, England: NFER Publishing, 1978.

Goldberg, D. Training family practice residents to recognize psychiatric disturbances. Final report, contract No. ADAMHA 278-78-0039 (DB), Washington, D.C., 1980.

Goldberg, I. D., Allen, G., Kessler, L. G., Carey, J. F., Locke, B. Z., & Cook, W. A. Utilization of medical services after short-term psychiatric therapy in a prepaid health plan setting. *Medical Care,* in press.

Goldberg, I. D., Krantz, G., & Locke, B. Z. Effect of a short-term outpatient psychiatric benefit on the utilization of medical services in a prepaid group practice medical program. *Medical Care*, 1970, 8, 419-428.

Goldman, H. H., Burns, B. J., & Burke, J. D. Integrating primary health care and mental health services: A preliminary report. *Public Health Reports*, 1980, 95, 535-539.

Hankin, J., & Oktay, J. S. *Mental disorder and primary medical care: An analytic review of the literature*. National Institute of Mental Health, Series D, No. 5, DHEW Publication No. (ADM) 78-661. Washington, DC: Government Printing Office, 1979.

Health Services Administration and the Alcohol, Drug Abuse and Mental Health Administration. Inter-agency agreement between HSA and ADAMHA to improve alcohol, drug abuse, and mental (ADM) health services in primary care and to use available service resources more effectively. Rockville, Maryland, 1980.

Hoeper, E. W., Nycz, G. R., Cleary, P. D., Regier, D. A., & Goldberg, I. D. Estimated prevalence of RDC mental disorder in primary medical care. *International Journal of Mental Health*, 1979, 8, 6-15.

Houpt, J. L., Orleans, C. S., George, L. K., & Brodie, H. K. H. The importance of mental health services to general health care. Cambridge, MA: Ballinger, 1979.

Jacobson, A. M., Regier, D. A., & Burns, B. J. Factors relating to the use of mental health services in a neighborhood health center. *Public Health Reports*, 1978, 93, 232-239.

Jones, K. R., & Vischi, T. R. Impact of alcohol, drug abuse and mental health treatment on medical care utilization: A review of the research literature. *Medical Care* (Supplement), 1979, 17.

Locke, B. Z. Patients, psychiatric problems, and nonpsychiatric physicians in a prepaid group practice medical program. *American Journal of Psychiatry*, 1966, 123, 207-210.

Locke, B. Z., Finucane, D. L., & Hassler, F. Emotionally disturbed patients under care of private nonpsychiatric physicians. *American Psychiatric Association: Psychiatric Research Report*, 1967, 22, 235-248.

Locke, B. Z., & Gardner, E. A. Psychiatric disorders among patients of general practitioners and internists. *Public Health Reports*, 1969, 84, 167-173.

Marks, J. N., Goldberg, D. P., & Hillier, V. F. Determinants of the ability of general practitioners to detect psychiatric illness. *Psychological Medicine*, 1979, 9, 337-353.

National Institute of Mental Health. Manpower systems development grant announcements. Rockville, MD: NIMH, Division of Manpower and Training Programs, 1979. (a)

National Institute of Mental Health. Mental health services manpower development and training grants announcements. Rockville, MD: NIMH, Division of Manpower and Training Programs, 1979. (b)

Parron, D. L., & Solomon, F. (Eds.). *Mental health services in primary care settings: Report of a conference, April 2-3, 1979*. DHHS Publication No. (ADM) 80-995. Washington, DC: Government Printing Office, 1980.

Parry, H. J., Balter, M. B., Mellinger, G. D., Cisin, I. N., & Manheimer, D. I. National patterns of psychotherapeutic drug use. *Archives of General Psychiatry*, 1973, 29, 769-783.

President's Commission on Mental Health. Report to the President. Washington, DC: Government Printing Office, 1978.

Regier, D. A. & Goldberg, I. D. National health insurance and the mental health services equilibrium. Paper presented at the annual meeting of the American Psychiatric Association, May 1976.

Regier, D. A., Goldberg, I. D., Kessler, L. G., & Burns, B. J. Overview. In D. A. Regier, I. D. Goldberg, & B. J. Burns (Eds.), *Use of health and mental health outpatient services in four organized health-care settings*. DHHS Publication No. (ADM) 80-859. Washington, DC: Government Printing Office, 1980.

Regier, D. A., Goldberg, I. D., & Taube, C. A. The de facto U.S. mental health services system. *Archives of General Psychiatry,* 1978, 35, 685-693.

Regier, D. A., & Rosenfeld, A. H. The report of the NIMH work group on mental health training of primary care providers. Rockville, Maryland, 1977.

Rosen, B. M., Locke, B. Z., Goldberg, I. D., & Babigian, H. M. Identification of emotional disturbance in patients seen in general medical clinics. *Hospital and Community Psychiatry,* 1972, 23, 364-370.

Shepherd, M. Mental health as an integrant of primary care. In D. L. Parron & F. Solomon (Eds.), *Mental health services in primary care settings: Report of a conference, April 2-3, 1979.* DHHS Publication No. (ADM) 80-995. Washington, DC: Government Printing Office, 1980.

Shepherd, M., Cooper, B., Brown, A. C., & Kalton, G. W. *Psychiatric illness in general practice.* London: Oxford University Press, 1966.

Vaillant, G. E. Natural history of male psychologic health: Effects of mental health on physical health. *New England Journal of Medicine,* 1979, 301, 1249-1254.

3

Coordinating Health and Mental Health Planning

Homer J. Hagedorn
Arthur D. Little, Inc.
Cambridge, Massachusetts

Introduction

As the 1980s get underway, coordination of mental and physical health planning in the United States is still in a stage of preliminary evolution. Generally, coordination does occur among various segments of the mental health delivery system, and it takes place under the auspices of agencies created under PL 93-641, the Health Planning and Resource Development Act of 1974. A good example of this kind of coordination would be a Health Systems Agency (HSA) task force in which county mental health officials, directors of substance abuse programs, psychiatric service chiefs from community hospitals, and board members or executive staff from federally funded community mental health centers work together in subcommittees staffed by the HSA to prepare or revise the mental health section of the HSA's Health System Plan.

Considerable amounts of constructive activity have come about in anticipation or recognition of the health planning amendments of 1979 (PL 96-79). Under Sections 1512 and 1513 of PL 93-641, as revised under these amendments, HSAs are required to include mental health expertise on their staffs, to include mental health representatives in governing bodies and executive committees, and to coordinate their activities with other substate planning agencies, including mental health planning agencies.

Mandated requirements for coordination constitute a push. The result of this push is memoranda of agreement, exchanges of liaison representatives, mutual document reviews, common memberships, and the creation of other shared channels and interconnections. What passes through these connections and channels, however, depends upon whether any shared attraction exists. There is always some degree of shared desire to take a comprehensive approach that will be able to overcome the shortcomings inherent in categorical service programs. Indeed, the desire to bring about adequately comprehensive solutions is the usual basis for mandating coordination in the first place. Coordination is supposed to make up for too much success in building categorical programs that subsequently do not work together.

At the level of local service delivery, there is still little indication of coordinated planning between family practice and other primary care physicians and mental health centers and clinics, or between acute care hospitals and facilities of the state mental health system. Nor are there many indications of state-level coordination of planning of mental and physical health services. Although there is surely a trend toward a "holistic" perspective and increasing willingness to accept and act on the importance of mental and emotional factors in physical illness, it is simply not on a holistic level that coordination is now occurring. The deep divisions in ideology, discrepancies in treatment priorities, and differences in economic interests that exist between so many private practice physicians and members of the mental health professions may for a long time continue to preclude their collaboration. On the other hand, the steady proliferation of HMOs, clinics, and group practices that to some extent bridge the gaps among provider personnel of various disciplines may make for swifter changes than heretofore seemed likely. Greater coordination could be the result if all parties continue to be placed under economic pressure by inflation, by continued efforts to contain health care costs, and by the licensing and certification of more physicians than are needed to satisfy demand.

Barriers to coordination between mental health planners and physical health planners are considerably less inhibiting than those among the service providers but are still real enough. In a recent study contracted by the Health Resources Administration, Arthur D. Little, Inc., in collaboration with its subcontractor, the Alpha Center for Health Planning, examined barriers and facilitators of coordination in nine states.[1] Much of the material in this chapter is drawn from that study, including the overview presented in this introduction.

Recent Coordination Efforts in
Physical and Mental Health Planning

In this section we will summarize the coordination efforts we encountered in the nine-state study just mentioned. During that work, we concluded that coordination is best thought of as a "process" rather than an administrative "condition." Accordingly, the summaries presented in this chapter describe projects that have waxed and waned, rather than structural arrangements achieved and maintained. Coordination may well lead to permanent results, such as durable changes in institutional procedures or policies, or long-lived cooperation among elements of the service delivery system. But the most effective coordination efforts we found were actually devised and experienced as very specific attempts to solve very concrete problems. For example, the Massachusetts Department of Mental Health and the Office of State Health Planning eventually found it possible to agree on a population-related standard for the number of psychiatric inpatient beds required in a health service area. They could agree as they began their work that there was no acceptable standard; they found they could agree on a mutually acceptable process for developing a standard. Many months later they arrived at a specific standard that is apparently acceptable, is currently in use, and will certainly provide a reasonably solid base whose foundations both parties understand. But the parties could *not* agree on general questions of priority and relationship, such as who might exercise what initiatives in the planning process. Their work was delayed by the unwillingness of one party or another to consent to steps that might ultimately be used to limit their authority. Thus, they quickly learned that it was essential to avoid discussions that brought to the surface, or implied, power and authority issues if they truly wanted to make progress. Very often getting specific was the easiest way, accordingly, to get anywhere in their discussion. Differences in perspectives, priorities, and opinions about the relative value and feasibility of quantitative standards could be honored only if concurrence on these broader matters were not made essential to the more specific negotiation and agreement they had determined to seek.

In one sense, there is nothing novel in this class of findings. Diplomatic, legal, and business negotiations have traditionally sought to be concrete in their representations whenever their primary objectives have been the settlement of material, as opposed to ideological, differences between independent parties. The novelty arises because it has been so easy to think of coordination as a way to straighten out problems about authority and the proper distribution—or concentration—of political power in public settings. The folly of using coordination to compensate for the excesses of categorical behavior precisely illustrates the point.

Coordinative processes paradoxically permit their practitioners to approach policy and authority problems only through piling up practical precedents. Where two organizations do not report directly to the same boss—and even in some cases when they do have the same immediate boss—there is obviously very little that can be done peaceably to bring about involuntary agreement between them. The consequence is that "coordination" in matters of substance is a lot more like voluntary agreement than it is a common acceptance of authority.

What happens when the attempt to coordinate is made? Let us summarize some relatively concrete attempts to solve immediate, tangible problems.

Massachusetts

The Massachusetts case mentioned earlier is one such case. The needs of the state health planners and the leadership of the Department of Mental Health were quite different. But at least one common problem existed. The number of applications for certificates of need from general hospitals for permission to establish acute psychiatric inpatient units was increasing in the mid-1970s. Economic pressures on general hospitals to reduce length of patient stay in all beds and to increase occupancy rates in general coincided with continuing decreases in demand for obstetrical services. Consequently, many general hospitals anticipated excessive bed capacity. The Department of Mental Health was concerned lest the Department of Health, including the state health planners, would respond to these applications for psychiatric beds without complete undersanding of public mental health programs and implications for the accessibility of mental health services to people without strong financial backing. The Department of Health was concerned that the Department of Mental Health's deinstitutionalization policies could threaten the Public Health Department's attempts to contain health care costs by controlling general hospital bed supply. The state health planners and HSA representatives developed a psychiatric bed standard without direct participation of state mental health officials. Pressure in 1976 from a higher level, the state's secretary of human services, to work together resulted in development of an interim standard rate for psychiatric beds per 100,000 being negotiated between the health planners in public health and mental health officials. But many issues went unresolved until specifics were tackled by a task force that included service providers, financial intermediaries and advocates, in addition to the health planners, mental health state administrators, the HSA representatives who had been involved in earlier stages of the process. This larger and more varied group, through ten subcommittees, slowly and painstakingly worked out commonly acceptable solutions to the following problems:

- definition of acute psychiatric units in general hospitals,

- definition of patients appropriate for acute inpatient psychiatric treatment,

- guidelines for determining size of acute psychiatric units in general hospitals,

- guidance on average length of stay for patients in acute inpatient psychiatric care,

- further definition of the psychiatric bed need formula,

- criteria for choosing general hospitals that could appropriately operate acute psychiatric inpatient units,

- agreed-upon method for using mental health catchment areas as health service area planning bases,

- criteria and procedure for placement of involuntary patients in general hospital acute psychiatric inpatient units,

- affiliation between acute psychiatric inpatient units in general hospitals and other mental health catchment area programs, and

- initial steps with respect to financial and economic considerations.

Requisite regulations were ultimately developed. Over 800 beds have been approved under the new standard.

The principles ultimately followed in gaining agreement on these difficult issues were:

- Recognize that the problem is owned by more than one agency, that it involves a variety of interests, and that it will be perceived very differently by different groups.

- Welcome everyone who is a party at interest into the developmental process to help formulate possible solutions and to help shape necessary negotiations.

- Make sure that a workable and adequate coalition develops to force the agreed-upon solution into practice.

- Use political and management authority when it is available to force reluctant parties to get involved.

- Avoid disputes over abstract issues. Admit that the collective interest and authority is insufficient to resolve these generic issues. Work hard to become specific and to identify negotiable specifics in order to move beyond objections that are voiced.

- Choose problems for coordinated action for which major parties at interest agree that there is an urgent need for practical solution and little or no possibility for ex parte solutions to be accepted.

Illinois

In Illinois, an active coordination effort has evolved around the Illinois Commission on Mental Health and Developmental Disabilities. Legislative enactment of the commission in 1975 was an important step in the process, but the preliminary work and political effort necessary to legislate the commission in the first place was also a major part of the effort. What is being attempted is a comprehensive coordination of federally mandated planning in over a dozen mental health, developmental disabilities, and substance abuse programs with the state legislative budgeting and appropriation process. Actually being coordinated by this planning process are the specific needs of numerous, sometimes competing, local programs. The incentive for local participation is the opportunity for funding under plans put in place and agreed to at local levels under the auspices of the HSAs. The goal of the coordinated process is to provide enough political advocacy and support to assure that the state appropriation bill emerges from the legislature with priorities recognizable at the local level.

But the starting point for what has so far been a six-year effort was nothing so grand or abstract as getting the state budget to respond to formalized human services planning. The starting point was a desire to reinstitute overall system planning as a function applicable to the Department of Mental Health and Developmental Disabilities: concretely, to set up a small planning staff governed by a joint executive branch and legislative commission. The first task of the staff was to inventory and describe what was required and being done under 14 different mandated, and relatively categorical, federal or state planning processes relevant to the department. The complexity and overlap of these mandated planning requirements, coupled with the question "How can you implement a plan anyway?" is what ultimately led to the attempt to link planning with the state budget and appropriations process. This concept was written into Illinois law in 1979, thus authoritatively establishing state mental health planning, state health planning of the mental health system under PL 93-641, and the preparation of the budget of the Department of Mental Health and Developmental Disabilities under one process.

It may require another year or more to demonstrate how much impact can be derived from coordinated planning and budgeting. Myriad different planning cycles, somewhat spotty initial acceptance of the idea, and the subtlety and complexity of incorporating planning considerations directly into political and administrative process have made for implementation difficulties. Nor has the leadership of all the federal programs involved been uniformly accepting—despite the existence since 1979 of a staff funded by the Federal Planning Reform Demonstration project. Much of the state-level leadership for the planning effort has been continuous and unremitting in its efforts. Slow turnover in the early leadership has been coupled with a continued infusion of new leaders sufficiently interested to sustain and review the effort and to broaden support for it at critical points.

The Illinois example illustrates the same principles that applied to the Massachusetts care plus some additional ones:

- It helps to have a state mandate for planning coordination to match the federal mandates.

- Skills in building networks and coalitions are essential for coordination on a broad scale.

- The role of continuing strong leadership is vital.

West Virginia

Another type of coordinated physical and mental health planning has been attempted in West Virginia. In this instance, the motivating forces appear to have been a desire to do the mandated federal planning with as much efficiency as possible, using minimum necessary manpower, and a desire to make the planning process a handmaiden to the total reorganization of health and mental health activities of the state government. In a state where relatively scanty private resources in health care necessitate a larger role for public health care service delivery agencies, the need for comprehensive rather than categorical approaches has had a great impact. Hence, statewide *behavioral* health planning was organized around the service taxonomy recognized in PL 93-641, rather than organ-centered, disease-specific, or service modality categories:

- health promotion and protection

- prevention and detection

- diagnosis and treatment

- habilitation; rehabilitation and maintenance

- support

Task forces organized to write behavioral health plan components around each of these subjects included representatives of the various categorical approaches in mental health and substance abuse, providers and consumers, and local and statewide interests. The fact that West Virginia has only one statewide health systems agency has enabled consolidation of the Health Systems Plan and the State Health Plan, one major step toward being able to use the West Virginia Behavioral Health Plan to satisfy all the federally mandated mental or behavioral health planning requirements as well as the mental health planning requirements under PL 93-641.

In the organization of the West Virginia Department of Health, the federal and state categorical programs are made subordinate to the Office of Community Services. State institutions for long-term care, acute care, mental illness, and mental retardation are grouped into the Office of Institutional Services. The third major component of the department is the Office of Health Planning and Evaluation. Thus, administrative integration among the categorical service delivery programs of the state, based on the type of service setting, becomes another available element in system linkage, and planning integration or coordination is facilitated by concentrating responsibilities for planning as clearly as possible within one comprehensive or holistic health planning office.

This approach to coordination might seem to be almost self-implementing and not at all sensitive to changes in the leadership cadre, since it can be presented in a highly conceptual and elegant fashion. It is, however, strongly subject to the vagaries associated with changes or temporary faltering in leadership. That is, an organizational model at the state level does not change the objectives, constituencies, attitudes, or scope of categorical program managers in federal service, or the constraints and priorities of those managing state or local projects of these categorical programs. Thus, even what seems to be a unified and sweeping rationalization of authority turns out to require a great deal of persuasiveness, persistence, and sheer gumption in the face of adversity. Like the other two attempts at planning coordination described earlier, the West Virginia effort has waxed, waned, and renewed itself at various times. At times its durability and its impact have both been in doubt. To have placed the success of the attempt completely beyond doubt would have required many low probability events;

the U.S. Congress and the West Virginia legislature acting in parallel, a broader and deeper federal commitment to coordination, continued tenure of the incumbent leadership of the West Virginia Department of Health and the administration of Governor Rockefeller, and new and highly collaborative attitudes arising in both the administrative and professional staffs of the categorical programs. It is the difficulty or impossibility of achieving simultaneous unanimity of tenure, policy, and priority or so many governing instrumentalities that explains the need and justifies the utility of coordination projects.

New Mexico

In New Mexico, the attempt was made in 1979 and 1980 to establish substate, regional technical advisory groups (TAGS) to provide unified local input to mental and physical health planning and review processes. The idea was generated in a joint task force including state behavioral health planners, state health planners, and HSA representatives. The TAGS were in fact established. However, their connections to both the state Behavioral Health Division and to the regional councils of the HSA resulted in more confusion and vagueness than could be coped with during the first year. Possibly, the TAGS could have successfully contended with developing their own priorities and establishing their own relationships with others. But the state Behavioral Health Division, which funded each TAG's part-time staff, needed to be sure that each regional TAG did not become an appendage of the HSA, because the HSA was outside state government and could have no responsibility for operating state-funded programs—including, apparently, developing plans and reviewing grant applications. But the HSA could accept the review of each TAG as HSA work only if the TAG was functioning as an HSA regional council subcommittee. In the short term, these two positions were perceived as irreconcilable. The TAGS could not or did not take the initiative that would be required to overcome the effects of these skeptical, if not mutually exclusive, viewpoints. The upshot, after over six months of operation, was a noticeable degree of frustration. TAG members had hoped that the TAG structure would simplify and shorten the review processes under state law and PL 93-641. Instead, the TAG seemed to be functioning as an additional level of review, which disappointed TAG members, who were sensitive to the shortage of well-trained people to serve on local review and planning bodies. The HSA and state health and mental health planners seemed to understand one another's positions well, but each wondered if the other was really constrained to take *only* the position each espoused, or whether more flexibility could have been shown. Given time, persistence, further negotiation, and continuity of committed leadership, the TAG concept could prove both feasible and useful in the New Mexico situation. Since the state and HSA officials tended to cite law and program policy as a justification for their respective positions, it is possible that the feasibility of the TAG structure will actually turn on the willingness of higher-level state and federal officials to allow practical coordinative devices like TAGS to function effectively.

Connecticut and Indiana

In Connecticut and Indiana, interesting attempts have been made to coordinate or consolidate mental health planning required of the HSA. In Connecticut, Regional Mental Health Boards, through contracts, assigned state and locally generated planning funds to the HSAs, so that the HSAs could conduct all of the technical planning processes connected with mental health planning in the region. However, this step did not imply that the Regional Mental Health Boards had ceded legal responsibilities. Since this arrangement permitted use of the mental health funds to generate some federal matching funds for the HSAs, the contracts greatly increased the amount and quality of professional planning that was affordable. In Indiana, analogous contracts have been stimulated by the state Department of Mental Health for many years. Most recently, the state has contracted with HSAs to conduct the technical side of the planning process, following a standardized format that has made compilation of the Mental Health Plan a very simple exercise. But in neither Connecticut nor Indiana have there yet been committed efforts to use coordinated planning activity to accomplish actual changes in the system of allocating resources to the health and mental health service delivery systems, nor have these states attempted to address specific controversial problems of service delivery. The Indiana system had been in operation more or less continuously since 1963 in a political environment not consistently hospitable to social planning. Perhaps this environment also explains the reluctance of the state legislature to continue funding the Department of Mental Health to pay for substate planning contracts when funds under Section 314 (d) of the Public Health Service Act became unavailable in 1980. In Connecticut's case, it is too early to predict the results of the locally consolidated planning process.

Florida

The case of coordinated planning in Florida is not dissimilar from Indiana and Connecticut. In Florida, NIMH awarded a grant to the Florida Council of Community Mental Health to train people in three specific health and mental health planning processes: needs assessment, planning resource development, and the health or mental health service project grant review process. Projects were carried out in different areas throughout the state, training staff and citizen members of the HSAs and the district mental health boards (DMHBs). The DMHBs in Florida are nonprofit citizen boards created through state legislation to conduct planning, allocate state and county funds to local-level provider agencies within each of the 11 districts throughout the state, and review and monitor these service provider agencies, primarily community mental health centers. For the most part, the HSAs in the state have coterminous boundaries with the state district structure, although there may be several DMHBs within a single HSA area.

The people involved with the DMHB and those involved in the HSAs generally knew each other prior to the advent of these training demonstrations. The training process, however, created an opportunity and a context in which they could work more closely. The utility of the training process was that it "credentialed" the process of coordination and provided a facilitative forum within which a developing relationship between the DMHBs and the corresponding HSA could be expedited and carried forward. In essence, a formalized third party intermediary, the training team brought people, interests, and skills together to work on substantive issues. For example, in one area they concentrated on developing common criteria and grant review procedures so each CMHC in the district would not have to go through separate, duplicative, yet somewhat different grant review processes with their DMHB and their respective HSA. The training process admitted to the legitimacy of both the DMHB and the HSA and did not try to change the relative power or authority of one vis-à-vis the other. As in Massachusetts, progress was able to be realized on specific, substantive issues.

Texas

Texas illustrates an explicit and overt attempt to build a statewide coalition of state and local interests to overcome the barriers to coordinated planning caused partly by a highly decentralized group of state agencies, each with some planning responsibilities in the areas of health and mental health. Texas, in comparison to many other states, could be characterized as having a government structure and process that leaves relatively greater authority in the State legislature than the executive branch. Furthermore, the decentralized nature of the executive branch created a situation where over a dozen agencies had some role in health and mental health planning. The results of these two facts, a strong legislature and a decentralized executive structure, led to the common understanding that the only real plan was the state legislative budget.

After grappling with the problems of coordination, leaders in several state agencies, primarily the state Departments of Health and Mental Health and Retardation decided to "get everybody together." A conference was organized and attended by over 300 persons representing state and local government agencies, as well as special interest and advocacy groups. The primary goal of the conference was to teach representatives about the details of the required planning processes, the technical intricacies mandated by the federal laws and regulations. Many participants hoped the conference would stimulate a process of coordinated planning that might ultimately take the form of linking federally mandated planning to the state budget process, not unlike efforts described earlier in our discussion of Illinois.

While the final verdict is out with respect to linking planning with the budget, the approach used in Texas is one method of dealing with the problems presented by multiple power centers having planning responsibilities. Certainly, the strategy used by Texas planners is a clear effort at coalition and consensus-building, in sharp contrast to our next and final example, where powerful but separate state agencies tried to deal with one another on questions of authority, going far beyond the negotiated resolution of specific, substantive issues.

California

Over a three-year period the California Department of Mental Health (DMH) and the California Office of Statewide Health Planning and Development (OSHPD) negotiated successfully with one another on specific issues, such as a manpower development grant and criteria for a new type of acute psychiatric care facility. They also had negotiated a memorandum of agreement that broadly endorsed the principle of coordinated planning and provided that each would share information with the other.

Then two requirements emerged which drove these two strong agencies toward one another and into overt conflict. By state law, the DMH had to develop a deinstitutionalization plan. At the same time, the OSHPD was identified as the new state agency for coordinating all federally mandated health planning requirements. Consequently, each agency was motivated to do a lot of planning *and* to maintain control over their own planning processes.

The OSHPD produced a state health plan that included a component chapter on mental health. For a number of reasons the DMH did not have its own plan in place, nor did it provide much input to the OSHPD mental health component plan. This lack of input also allowed the DMH to divorce itself from the OSHPD component plan.

This was the atmosphere that existed at the time the OSHPD proposed a revision in the memorandum of agreement. But now neither agency seemed capable of negotiating their principal differences in at least two respects. First, would the DMH be the single major source for the mental health component of the state health plan, or just one of several major sources? Second, what would be the respective roles of the DMH and the OSHPD in overseeing the coordination of mental health planning at the substate and county level: the OSPHD-HSA combination or the DMH and an emergent DMH regional structure? There were a variety of real management control and fiscal concerns on the part of county-owned and operated mental health service agencies that further amplified the growing disagreement between the OSHPD and the DMH and that tended to create alliances with one side or the other at the local level.

The major point to be made is that both agencies become locked into a relationship dominated by their concerns about ultimate authority and the possibility of being placed in a subordinate role if they accepted new language proposed by the other in a memorandum of understanding. Once the relationship became permeated by such concerns, coordination of any substantive kind became much more difficult. We do not intend to convey a sharp chronological shift from cooperation to confrontation. Rather, as the relative mix of substantive versus power issues shifted gradually to a greater emphasis on power, there was a gradual increase in the difficulties of achieving even substantive agreements. Though substantive agreements were possible, they become more complicated whenever they were tinged with issues of power.

The Process-Outcome Balance

In many states, the emphasis in coordination of mental and physical health planning has been structural, relational, and administrative. The goal has been to achieve a coordinated planning process and to leave to this process the elucidation of specific, substantive planning goals and system policies. Such an emphasis on achieving procedural coordination is not necessarily wrong, but it is different from any attempt to use coordination as a way of containing costs, improving accessibility or quality, changing the allocation of public funds among the service delivery sectors, overcoming the negative effects of excessively categorical operations, or supporting a deinstitutionalization policy. It is the contention of this chapter that the most important opportunity "coordination" can offer is the opportunity to grapple effectively with matters of substance that are not within the purview of any one existing structure. The author concedes a prejudice for coordination efforts that are designed to influence and change concrete problems of the service delivery system. Coordination merely for the sake of efficient compliance, or mutual communication, or minimizing procedural duplication can be valuable, but it seems less important. However, as earlier stated, attempts to change substance also provide opportunities to confront abstract and insoluble issues about power and authority.

Training, networking, and coalition-building can readily produce substantive changes, though each may be delimited in scope. But incremental changes may be adequate once some momentum is maintained. Coordination through power brokering can also work to produce system change but under a limited number of circumstances. It may work when a superordinate authority, such as the state's governor, makes the decision and provides the resources to centralize planning and allocation authority. Coordination may also work when an emergent public consensus transcends the differences among agencies and their associated ideological positions, or when a coalition- and consensus-building process succeeds in bringing pressure upon government officials.

Generally, coordinated planning remains a weak counterforce to the older, more prevalent and entrenched categorical planning, funding, and service delivery system. However, with greater awareness of the optional approaches and their likely outcomes and side effects and with increasing skill in the management of the coordination process we may hope to advance the power and precision of coordinated planning.

Note

1. Contract No. HRA 232-79-0090. James A. Stockdill, then Acting Associate Administrator of HRA, originated the study; Isabel Price, Ph.D., was Project Officer. Project team members included Alexandra Walcott, Helen Schauffler, Kenneth Beck, Ann Venable, Boyd Palmer (Alpha Center), and Alan Bayer (Alpha Center). The author served as project director.

4

The Tangled Web of
Clinical and Epidemiological Evidence

Eric N. Goplerud
Northside Community Mental Health Center,
Tampa, Florida

Health planners have grown increasingly concerned about the nature and scope of mental health problems in primary health care settings. Although the frequency of psychiatric disturbance in primary care settings is not known with certainty, evidence suggests that 30-60% of patients in general hospital units, and 50-80% of general practice outpatients suffer from emotional distress of sufficient severity to pose problems in medical management (Houpt, Orleans, George, & Brodie, 1980; Schwab, Bell, Warheit, & Schwab, 1970). Psychosocial factors appear prominent in three primary health care populations: (1) patients with exclusively psychiatric disorders; (2) patients with organic diseases for whom psychosocial factors play a role in the predisposition, initiation, or mediation of the illness; and (3) patients who suffer from psychological disturbances in reaction to or as a result of their organic illnesses. A few voices have also raised concerns about the prevalence and treatment of medically ill patients in the mental health sector (Koranyi, 1972, 1977, 1979; Kampmeier, 1977; Rossman, 1969).

On a clinical level, health and mental health do not separate easily into two distinct domains. Repeatedly researchers have demonstrated that persons with medical problems are frequently found in psychiatric care settings, and persons with emotional problems are treated more frequently within the primary health care sector than in all mental health clinics in the United States. In the course of a year, the mental health sector treats only 21 percent of all persons estimated to have emotional disorders (Regier, Goldberg, & Taube, 1978). Fifty-four percent are seen in the outpatient health sector and another six percent are seen jointly in mental health and health settings. General hospitals and nursing homes care for an additional three percent. The remainder either receive no treatment or remain unaccounted for.

Modifiable lifestyle and behavioral patterns have been implicated in five of the six leading causes of death in the United States (diseases of the heart and blood vessels, accidents, diabetes mellitis, and cirrhosis of the liver) and in the major causes of disability (cardiovascular diseases, chronic obstructive pulmonary disease, and accidents; see Gori & Richter, 1978; Houpt et al., 1979). Another behavioral problem of considerable concern is the pervasive noncompliance on the part of 15 to 50 percent of persons who receive medical advice or are placed on medical regimens (Houpt et al., 1979). Researchers have also demonstrated associations between stressful life events, chronic stressful conditions, and social support on the one hand and the onset, duration, and course of a wide variety of medical disorders on the other (Biegel et al., 1980; Depue, 1980; Dohrenwend & Dohrenwend, 1969; Goplerud, 1979, 1980; Rabkin & Struening, 1976).

Psychosocial and physiological factors also appear inseparable in mental health practice. Careful physical and laboratory examination of psychiatric outpatient (Koranyi, 1972, 1979), emergency (Browning, Miller, & Tyson, 1974; Leeman, 1975), and inpatient populations (Maguire & Granville-Grossman, 1968) have disclosed concurrent psychiatric and medical disorders in 30-50 percent of patients. For a significant minority, organic pathology proves to be the sole and exclusive cause of presenting emotional complaints. Psychiatrists, who serve as one bridge between health and mental health sectors, failed to properly diagnose underlying organic illnesses in about half of the psychiatric patients studied (Koranyi, 1972, 1979; Maguire & Granville-Grossman, 1968). Another concern raised about the medical status of emotionally disturbed patients focuses on the elevated mortality rates found among psychiatric inpatients (Kolb, 1976; Kampmeier, 1977), outpatients (Koranyi, 1977; Rorsman, 1974), and deinstitutionalized patients (Goplerud, 1979). Greater than expected mortality from all causes—suicide, accidents, and natural causes—have been found repeatedly in hospitalized and outpatient psychiatric populations.

Finally, a sophisticated literature has emerged demonstrating the effects of stress and social support on the onset, severity, and chronicity of psychiatric disorders (Depue, 1980; Dohrenwend & Dohrenwend, 1969; Rabkin, 1980). This chapter will review the extent to which mental health and somatic health are enmeshed at the clinical level in both the primary health care sector and the specialized mental health care sector.

Community Prevalence of
Mental and Somatic Illnesses

Community surveys suggest considerable overlap between emotional and physical disorders. Schwab and his colleagues (1979) assessed the emotional and physical status of a stratified community sample in Alachua County, Florida. Using self-report questionnaires, they estimated that 28.1 percent of the population had emotional problems which could benefit from psychiatric interventions, 39 percent reported one or more physical illnesses, and 26 percent reported suffering frequently from one or more conditions in which psychological and biological factors jointly play a role, such as headaches, indigestion, constipation, nervous stomach, hypertension, asthma, peptic ulcer, and colitis. When Schwab et al. analyzed the concurrency of disorders, they found almost 10 percent of their sample reported all three kinds of disorders: emotional, somatic, and psychosomatic. Another eight percent reported both psychosomatic and physical disorders, and 2.6 percent reported emotional and psychosomatic disorders. Older respondents, blacks, females, the poor, and persons either divorced, separated, or widowed were disproportionately represented among those with concurrent illnesses (Schwab et al., 1979).

Although these results point to an impressive challenge to the primary health and mental health sectors, the absence of independent physical and laboratory validation of self-reported symptoms and the questionable validity and reliability of the symptom categories employed in the questionnaire limit the generalizability of the study. The limitations are especially problematic in the whole concept of classic psychosomatic conditions (Kaplan, Freedman, & Sadock, 1980; Weiner, 1977).

The limitations of Schwab et al.'s study were largely overcome in another epidemiological study which found very similar results (Eastwood & Trevelyan, 1972; Eastwood, 1975). A random sample of persons aged 40-64 who were registered with a group general medical practice in a London suburb were invited to participate in a health screening project. Medical and psychological status data were obtained on over 1400 persons through a self-report questionnaire of physical and psychiatric symptoms, the Cornell Medical Index (CMI), physical and laboratory tests, and a physical examination by a general practitioner. A sample of persons with high psychological distress scores on the CMI were matched on various sociodemographic dimensions with persons reporting low psychological distress, and both groups were interviewed "blind" by a psychiatrist using a standardized diagnostic interview schedule (Goldberg, Cooper, Eastwood, Kedward, & Shepherd, 1970). Eastwood and Trevelyan (1972) found that persons with diagnosable psychiatric disorders (5.1 percent of all males and 17.7 percent of all females) suffered from more major physical illnesses and more major psychosomatic conditions than did matched nonpsychiatrically disturbed controls. Both male and female cases had higher than expected rates of coronary heart disease, cardiovascular disease, and chronic lung disease. Psychiatrically disturbed males, but not females, also suffered from higher rates of minor psychosomatic conditions and minor physical illnesses than did nondisturbed controls.

Later we will focus on the prevalence of emotional and physical problems in patient groups in primary health and mental health settings. However, the advantage of focusing on community prevalence of physical, psychiatric, and psychosomatic conditions is to highlight the widespread entanglement of psychiatric and physical symptomatology. Also, the overlapping physical and psychiatric symptoms foreshadow the diagnostic and treatment confusion which has occurred in settings which focus exclusively on either the patients' health or mental health status. Clearly, for many people a treatment orientation solely focused on somatic pathology or psychological dynamics will fail to treat their problems in an adequate, comprehensive fashion.

Health Status in Mental Health Settings

The few studies investigating the concurrence of physical and emotional disorders in psychiatric populations have uncovered a thorny problem for mental health settings. Patients in mental health settings have higher than expected mortality from all causes, high morbidity rates for a variety of serious medical disorders, and, among a significant minority of patients, undetected physical illnesses which can account completely for their emotional symptomatology. Furthermore, mental health clinicians appear to frequently misinterpret or overlook symptoms of physical pathology in their patients.

Koranyi (1972) raised many of these issues in a preliminary study of 100 consecutive admissions to an outpatient psychiatric clinic. A very thorough medical and psychiatric screening revealed that half of those referred to the clinic had major, and often multiple major, physical illnesses. In 10 percent of the referrals, previously undetected physical pathology proved to be the only possible cause of presenting emotional complaints. A sequel to this study, scrutinizing 2070 consecutive admissions to the same outpatient clinic, confirmed the earlier findings (Koranyi, 1979). Each referral to the clinic received a complete physical examination, laboratory workup, psychiatric status interview, a brief psychological test battery, and a social history interview on intake. Costs of intake screening were underwritten by the Canadian National Health Service.

As in the preliminary report, Koranyi found a high rate of major physical illnesses which had active symptoms requiring medical treatment and which were cause for concern on medical grounds. Almost half of the physical illnesses had not been detected by referring sources. This problem of missed diagnoses was particularly pronounced in referrals from social agencies and self-referrals, but even psychiatrists and nonpsychiatric physicians failed to diagnose a third of the physical illnesses in patients they referred. Also, as in Koranyi's earlier study, almost one person in ten seeking psychiatric treatment suffered from a physical illness which alone was the cause of the psychological disturbance. The most frequently undiagnosed causal condition was diabetes mellitus. A similiar finding was also reported in inpatient psychiatric settings by Waitzkin (1966a, 1966b). Major physical illnesses aggravated or were intimately related to an otherwise independent psychiatric condition in 25 percent of all intakes. Major medical illnesses and psychiatric disorders coexisted independently in 15 percent of this sample (Koranyi, 1979).

Outpatient psychiatric clinics are not the only mental health settings in which patients' physical and psychiatric pathology overlap. In a six-month follow-up study of persons receiving emergency psychiatric treatment in a general hospital emergency room, more than double the expected hospitalization rate for medical reasons was found (Browning, Miller, & Tyson, 1974). On the basis of clinical experience, Leeman (1975) estimated that half of all emergency room admissions suffer from emotional distress which needs attention. However, very few present distinctive psychiatric clinical pictures, and most show mixed somatic and emotional symtomology. Dismissing the medical disorders of psychiatric emergencies, as the complaints of "crocks" and "GOMERS" (Get Out Of My Emergency Room), as such patients are sometimes called by staff, can lead to fatal consequences (Leeman, 1975; Koranyi, 1975).

Low rates of detecting physical illness in persons presenting acute psychiatric symptomatology has also been reported on inpatient psychiatric units. Maguire and Granville-Grossman (1968) found that 33.5 percent of 200 consecutive first admissions to a general hospital psychiatric unit had significant physical illnesses. As in the other studies of psychiatric populations, one half of these physical illnesses had not been previously detected.

Another indication of the cruicial significance of health status among psychiatric populations is the consistently high mortality rate found in both inpatient and outpatient groups (Goplerud, 1979, Hoenig & Hamilton, 1966; Kampmeier, 1977; Koranyi, 1977; Rorsman, 1974). In the past, reports of high mortality among psychiatric inpatients could be generally attributed to the peculiar role of state mental hospitals as the final repositories of the old, frail, sick, and impoverished (Goplerud, 1979; Kolb, 1976). However, even the most recent reports continue to find excessive mortality in all three major categories: suicide, accidents, and natural causes (Goplerud, 1979; Koranyi, 1977; Rorsman, 1974). Koranyi (1977), in a three-year follow-up study, found the mortality rate among psychiatric outpatients to be double that of the general population. Over four-fifths of those who died during the follow-up period suffered from major physical illnesses at the time of admission. In more than a third of the mortalities, the physical diagnosis was missed or insufficiently evaluated by the referring medical physician. Goplerud (1979) has also shown that the combination of physical frailty and psychiatric illness is correlated with extremely high mortality within the first three months following deinstitutionalization of elderly state hospital patients. High mortality rates among psychiatric patients underlines the necessity for providing comprehensive, ongoing medical and psychological assessment of patients in mental health settings.

Problems with Accurate Diagnosis

If physical pathology is as prevalent in mental health settings as the preceding section implies, why is it so often missed by clinicians? There appear to be problems on both sides of the couch.

Kampmeier (1977), a physician with 33 years of experience in the medical clinic of a large state hospital, outlined the problems he frequently encountered with psychiatric inpatients: (1) Patients frequently provide inadequate and unreliable medical histories; (2) they are often uncooperative with physical examinations; (3) they may fail to report significant symptoms or report a confusing mixture of real and delusional symptoms; and (4) they may be noncompliant or resistant to medical regimens. In a six-month study of consecutive referrals to the medical clinic, verbal information from the patient was helpful in reaching a diagnosis and treatment plan in only 10 percent of referrals (Kampmeier, 1977). Physical examination or observation was thought to contribute to diagnosis in 57 percent of patients. Numerous problems were encountered in performing examinations, especially with combative patients. Abstract information, primarily laboratory tests, provided diagnostic information in 58 percent of referrals. Finally, the glaring gaps and available bits of data, Kampmeier reported, are cemented into a diagnosis and treatment plan "by experience and a dash of intuition" (Kampmeier, 1977).

The complexity of the task of unraveling presenting psychological symptomatology and underlying organic pathology is demonstrated in a painstaking monograph by Davison and Bagley (1969). In their review of nearly 800 studies, these authors describe the differential diagnosis, pathogenesis, treatment, and prognosis of schizophrenic-like psychoses associated with organic disorders of the CNS. They conclude that an organic CNS disorder occurs in a substantial minority of patients with a diagnosis of schizophrenia, and that in most cases the organic disorder is a sufficient cause of the psychotic symptoms. Suspicion of CNS lesions or organic pathology should be entertained particularly in childhood schizophrenic-like psychoses and probably in psychoses among elderly, Davison and Bagley concluded. Specific organic disorders which mimic schizophrenia include epilepsy, cerebral trauma, cerebral tumor, encephalitides, basal ganglia disorders, nervous tissue degeneration, cardiovascular disorders, and metabolic and toxic CNS disorders (Davison & Bagley, 1969).

In a related vein, Hänninen (1978), a behavioral toxicologist, has demonstrated marked psychological and behavioral deterioration in workers exposed to such industrial chemicals as organic solvents, carbon monoxide, pesticides and heavy metals. Some of the effects of long term exposure to industrial chemicals produce CNS effects which mimic psychopathology. Other researchers have shown relationships between psychological symptoms and medications, especially corticosteroids, some antihypertensives, and psychotropics (Barchas, Berger, Claranell, & Elliot, 1977; Shader, 1972), noise (McLean & Tarnopolsky, 1977), shift work (NIOSH, 1976) and a variety of environmental factors in the workplace (Cooper & Payne, 1978).

Compounding the problems of accurate diagnosis, some organic diseases exhibit primarily or solely psychological symptoms in their early stages. These organic disorders appear repeatedly in studies of patients who initially received psychiatric diagnoses but who are later found to have organic diseases (Koranyi, 1972, 1977, 1979; Lipowski, 1975; Martin, 1980; Palarea, 1965; Rossman, 1969; Schwab, 1970). Psychiatric symptoms and organic diseases or conditions which cause them are listed in Table 4.1.

Rossman (1969) emphasized that diagnostic error occurs most easily when careful physical examinations and medical histories are not done, when patients suffer from rare organic conditions, or when patients are physically asymptomatic in prodromal stages of an illness and present only

TABLE 4.1   Psychiatric Symptoms and Organic Diseases

Depression	Affective, Organic, and Mixed Psychoses	Schizophrenia	Neurotic Disorders
Carcinoma of all sorts, particularly pancreatic	Systemic lupus erythematosis	Limbic system lesions	Porphyria
Viral infections	Corticosteroid therapy	Intracranial tumors	Hypoglycemia
Hypothyroidism (myxedema)		Temporal lobe epilepsy	Hyperthyroidism
Hyperparathyroidism/ hypoparathyroidism		Amphetamine and atabrine intoxication	Thiamine insufficiency
Parkinsonism		Addison's disease	Pheochromocytomia
Rheumatoid arthritis			Subdural hematoma
Adrenal cortical insufficiency			
Pernicious anemia			
Reserpine therapy			
Corticosteroid therapy			

psychiatric symptoms. Koranyi's (1979) careful analysis of undetected physical illnesses specifically highlights Rossman's third point. He found that five percent of his outpatient sample suffered from diabetes mellitus. Since erectile impotence in males occurs in early, otherwise asymptomatic stages of the illness, undetected diabetes may frequently be the cause of secondary psychiatric and marital problems.

Organizational, professional, and ideological factors in mental health settings also contribute to missed diagnoses of physical pathology. Later chapters in this book will review these factors and alternative solutions in greater detail. However, certain major problems will be noted here briefly.

Many mental health clinicians lack medical training. Psychological and psychiatric textbooks (e.g., Kaplan et al., 1980) pay attention only to psychological reactions to physical diseases and to psychosocial precursors of psychosomatic diseases. Furthermore, those mental health staff with greatest direct client contact, such as nurses aides, orderlies, and mental health workers, have the least medical and psychological training (U.S. DHEW., 1966).

A further problem is the tendency to interpret somatic symptoms as indicators of psychopathology rather than as signs of organic pathology (Kampmeier, 1977). Since physical complaints are very frequently presented by patients with clear psychiatric disorders, such a diagnostic bias can be expected. A corresponding but reverse bias in primary health settings, we shall see later, produces high rates of missed psychiatric diagnoses. Curiously, in some cases missed organic pathology responds to psychological treatment procedures. Hyperthyroidism, which typically presents with anxiety, affective lability, and sleep disturbance, may be diagnosed as bipolar affective disorder. Lithium, the treatment of choice for bipolar affective disorder, also suppresses thyroid activity, leading to a decrease in circulating thyroid and a reduction of "psychological" symptoms (Kline & Simpson, 1973).

To summarize, the evidence reviewed so far indicates that many of the patients in mental health settings suffer from physical illnesses which occur jointly with psychiatric disorders. For some patients, organic pathology, which is frequently undetected by mental health clinicians, totally accounts for their psychiatric symptoms. At this point it is reasonable to inquire whether similar overlap of organic and psychiatric pathologies occurs in primary health care settings.

Mental Health Status in Primary Care Settings

Emotional distress is practically ubiquitous among patients in primary health care settings. A typical report (Schwab, 1970) found that more than three-fourths of the patients studied in a general hospital medical ward complained of irritability, psychomotor retardation, anxiety, tension, and somatic preoccupation. Over half reported fatigue, insomnia, and depression. While such surveys indicate the high prevalence of emotional distress among primary care patients (see also Goldberg et al., 1970; Hoeper, Nycz, & Cleary, 1979; Shepherd, Cooper, Brown, & Kalton, 1966), there are three groups of patients for whom emotional distress is especially problematic: (1) patients with purely psychiatric disorders treated exclusively by primary care providers; (2) patients with organic disorders in which psychosocial factors play some part in the predisposition, initiation, or mediation of the illness; and (3) patients whose psychological symptoms are a reaction to or a result of an organic disease process.

Primary Psychiatric Disorders in Health Settings

Although the proportion of patients in primary care settings with primary psychiatric disorders (PPD) is small compared with total caseloads, the volume of service is great compared with that provided in the specialized mental health sector (Regier et al., 1978). Estimates of the prevalence of PPD and the volume of service provided vary with case identification methods, research settings, sociodemographic characteristics of patient populations, and sampling procedures (Hankin and Oktay, 1979). Most studies of primary care populations place the prevalence of PPD between 10 and 20 percent of all patients seen in a year and the incidence of new PPD at 3 to 7 percent each year (Hankin & Oktay, 1979; Houpt et al., 1979; WHO, 1973).

The actual prevalence of PPD in primary care practices is difficult to accurately determine. The most conservative case identification method relies on routine diagnostic reporting by primary care physicians. Studies in the United States have reported that at some time during the year between 4.2 and 29 percent of all adult primary care outpatients receive psychiatric diagnoses (Hankin & Oktay, 1979). The National Ambulatory Medical Care Survey (NAMCS) of all U.S. office-based physicians found a primary diagnosis of PPD recorded in 2.1 percent of visits to all nonpsychiatric physicians.

Using primary care physicians to identify PPD in the health sector probably undercounts true prevalence. Studies which have compared primary care physicians' with psychiatrists' diagnoses of general medical practice samples find that between one-third and one-half of the patients with PPD escape the notice of the primary care physician (Eastwood, 1975; Goldberg & Blackwell, 1970; Hoeper et al., 1979). Also, the reliability and validity of physicians' diagnoses have been questioned by evidence that variations in PPD diagnostic rates correlate with reported interest in psychiatry and previous training in psychotherapy (Shepherd et al., 1966).

Psychiatrists' diagnoses of PPD in general practice screening studies have been used as the yardstick for calculating the specificity and sensitivity of other case identification methods. Using standardized diagnostic interviews, which improve interrater and intrarater reliability, psychiatrists have found rates of mental disorder among outpatient adult samples between 11.6 and 26.7 percent (Hankin & Oktay, 1979; Hoeper et al., 1979; Regier, 1980).

However, it is difficult to determine in these surveys whether persons receiving psychiatric diagnoses also have coexisting physical diseases or whether the PPD is the sole condition for which patients are receiving treatment. Also, a question of the reliability of psychiatrists' judgment must be raised in light of the data reviewed in the previous section of this chapter.

The highest rates of psychiatric disturbance have been reported in non-psychiatric wards of general hospitals. Houpt and his colleagues reviewed three studies which report diagnosable psychiatric entities in 66.8 to 86 percent of ward residents (Houpt et al., 1979). Such high rates probably reflect patients' psychological reactions to organic disease and situational stress responses to hospitalization. Purely psychiatric disorders, particularly somatoform disorder, generalized anxiety disorder, and unipolar affective disorder, may account for an undefined number of disturbed inpatients (Kaplan et al., 1980). Researchers, using rigorous research diagnostic criteria, have not yet investigated the prevalence of PPD in general hospital wards.

Studies of children who exhibit emotional and behavioral disorders are relatively rare in primary health care settings. Jacobson and his colleagues (1980) reported on physician-recorded diagnostic rates for children under 18 in four organized health settings. Between 3.3 and 10.1 percent of all children attending the clinics received a psychiatric diagnosis at some point during the three-month study. When all enrolled patients, both clinic attenders and nonattenders, were included, the estimated annual prevalence of emotional or behavioral disorders ranged from 2.2 to 8.2 percent (Jacobson et al., 1980).

To some extent, prevalence rates reflect economic and demographic characteristics of the patient populations at risk. One of the most consistent findings in epidemiological research is the strong inverse relationship between socioeconomic class and psychopathology (Dohrenwend & Dohrenwend, 1969; Hankin & Oktay, 1978; Houpt et al., 1979). Education, another class correlate, is inversely related to emotional disorder. Also, studies in the general community, and in primary health care settings, have found that divorced, separated, and widowed persons are at increased risk for PPD (Dohrenwend & Dohrenwend, 1969; Houpt et al., 1979; Schwab et al., 1979). Relationships of PPD to age, race, sex, or religion remain unclear.

Although patients' sociodemographic characteristics, and hence risk for PPD, may vary widely from one primary care setting to another, a rough diagnostic distribution of PPD can be attempted. Probably the most methodologically sophisticated assessment of primary psychiatric diagnoses in a U.S. general medical practice was reported by Hoeper and his associates (1979, 1980), who documented the prevalence of psychiatric disorders among the patients of a large multispecialty group practice serving a town of

17,000 and its rural surrounding areas. Consecutive clinic patients were assessed by a psychiatrist using Research Diagnostic Criteria (RDC) in a standardized interview format, the Schedule of Affective Disorder-Schizophrenia (SADS-L). Weighting procedures were employed to statistically control for oversampling of high clinic utilizers and seasonal effects. Using RDC psychiatric diagnoses, Hoeper estimated the weighted annual prevalence of PPD to be 26.7 percent. Specifically, prevalence rates of depressive disorders (major, minor, and subsyndromal) was 19.9 percent, phobic disorder was 5.8 percent, and generalized anxiety disorder was 1.6 percent (Hoeper, 1980; Hoeper et al., 1979). Prevalence rates of other diagnostic categories was one percent or below. This high prevalence rate of depressive disorders has been reported also by most other diagnostic studies. Based on a review of 11 studies assessing PPD diagnostic distributions in primary care settings, Houpt and his colleagues (1979) state that "depression does appear to be the number one emotional disorder encountered in general medical practice" (p.25).

Characteristic PPD Symptomatology

It should not be surprising that the most common PPD diagnoses in general medical practices are depressive disorder, phobic disorder, and generalized anxiety disorder. Characteristic symptoms in each disorder include pronounced somatic distress and vegetative signs which may mimic other illnesses and produce confusion on the part of both physician and patient. Depressive disorders frequently exhibit somatic disturbances which include altered or disrupted sleep patterns, marked weight loss or gain, changes in psychomotor activity, and somatic preoccupation (Depue, 1980; Goplerud et al., in press). Comparing depressed patients with matched, psychiatrically normal controls, a recent longitudinal study found significantly higher levels of somatic concern, a greater number of somatic symptoms about a greater number of organ systems, more frequent self-medication with over-the-counter drugs, and more frequent use of prescription medication among the depressed persons, and particularly among dysthymic cases (Goplerud, Depue, Slater, & Fisher, in press). All subjects were medically screened at the beginning of the study, and none exhibited physical pathology. Jacobs, Gogelson, and Charles (1968) suggest that physicians should entertain the possibility of undetected chronic or intermittent depressive disorder in patients with recurrent somatic complaints and medical histories which include frequent clinical tests on multiple organ systems.

Generalized anxiety disorder and phobic disorder exhibit striking signs and symptoms which overlap with cardiovascular disorders. Panic attacks, which occur in both anxiety and phobic disorders, are discrete periods of sudden onset in which patients experience intense apprehension, fearfulness, or terror often associated with feelings of doom. Symptomatically, patients complain of violent heart palpitations, facial flush, pains in the chest—either sharp or constricting—respiratory difficulties, and a sense of dizziness, weakness, and faintness (Kaplan et al., 1980). In generalized anxiety disorder, where anxiety is a chronic condition, complaints of gastro-intestinal symptoms are common, as are chronic muscle contraction head-aches, sleep disturbance, easy fatigability during the day, and autonomic hyperactivity. Differential diagnosis of anxiety disorder and coronary artery disease must be made on the basis of laboratory and physical findings, as reports of concurrent anxiety disorder and coronary artery disease, though rare, have been published (Kaplan et al., 1980).

Finally, there is a small but well-known class of patients with somato-form disorders, a condition defined by DSM-III as "recurrent and multiple somatic complaints for which medical attention is sought; they are not apparently due to any physical illness, begin before early adulthood (prior to age 25) and have a chronic but fluctuating course." Estimates of the preva-lence of somatoform disorder (previously called hysteria or Briquet's syn-drome) are sketchy, but best figures using patient groups suggest a preva-lence of no more than one to two percent of women and below one percent in males (Woodruff, Goodwin, & Guze, 1974). The range of symptoms is very wide, and patients frequently report large numbers of symptoms which are distributed throughout all or nearly all organ systems. Chronic pain is promi-nent, especially headaches and chest, abdominal, back, and joint pains (Woodruff et al., 1974). Though relatively uncommon, these patients do overutilize primary health care services, are difficult to engage in psycho-therapy, and have a poor prognosis (Kaplan et al., 1980; Woodruff et al., 1974). One important caveat: Hysterical conversion disorders are most com-monly precipitated by neurological disorders. McKegney (1967) reported that 68 of 144 patients referred for psychiatric consultation because of con-version symptoms had preexisting or coexisting organic diseases.

PPD in Primary Care: Grounds for Concern

There are several reasons for concern that more than twice as many persons in the United States who have psychiatric disorders are treated in outpatient primary care settings than are treated in specialized mental health settings.

First, primary care physicians appear to underdetect and/or under-diagnose psychiatric disorders in their patients. At the extreme end, Hoeper et al. (1979) found that primary care physicians detected only three of 100 true cases of PPD when psychiatric diagnoses of patients were determined independently using research diagnostic criteria (RDC) and structured interview schedules. Other studies (Eastwood, 1975; Goldberg & Blackwell, 1970) have found rates of underdiagnosis between 33 and 50 percent. Underdiagnosis of PPD may contribute to the high reported rates of clinical tests, exploratory surgery, and nonpsychotropic drug treatment found among these patients (Goplerud et al., in press; Houpt et al., 1979; Kaplan et al., 1980; Woodruff et al., 1974).

Emotionally disturbed patients are referred very infrequently to mental health settings. Only 5 to 10 percent of identified PPD cases in primary care practices are referred (Eastwood, 1975; Hankin & Oktay, 1979; Houpt et al., 1979), although rates vary widely among individual physicians (Shepherd et al., 1966). Chemotherapy is the primary mode of treatment for identified PPD in primary care settings (67 percent of PPD visits; see Balter, 1973; Brown, Regier, & Balter, 1978; WHO, 1973). The appropriateness of primary care physicians' use of psychotropic drugs has been questioned, as has physicians' knowledge of drug interactions, side effects, and dose regulation (WHO, 1973).

Brief psychotherapy may also take place in about 22 percent of primary care visits, but time pressures on physicians limit the length of such sessions (Hankin & Oktay, 1979; Houpt et al., 1979). The average length of all primary care visits is about 13 minutes. One study found that PPD patients spend, on the average, 3.2 minutes more per visit to a nonpsychiatric physician than do patients not having a PPD diagnosis (Burns, Orso, Jacobsen, Leet, & Goldner, 1977). Not a single study has systematically investigated the clinical effectiveness of such brief physician-rendered therapy, nor has one compared clinical outcome from such interventions with other forms of psychotherapy.

Psychiatrically disturbed patients use about twice as many medical services as do nonpsychiatrically disturbed patients (Jones & Vischi, 1979). High utilization rates are found whether primary physician diagnoses of PPD or independent RDC diagnoses are used (Eastwood, 1975; Hankin & Oktay, 1979; Hoeper et al., 1979; Jones and Vischi, 1979). Since psychotherapy reduced the subsequent utilization of outpatient, inpatient, and laboratory services among patients with PPD in almost all studies (see Jones & Vischi, 1979), underdiagnosis of PPD may be producing an unnecessary drain on the patients' and the health sector's resources. Further investigation of the impact of effective diagnosis and treatment of PPD in primary care settings on use of health resources is clearly imperative.

In summary, the factors outlined in this chapter highlight the overlapping clinical domains of health and mental health care and the focal role primary physicians play in the treatment of psychiatric disorder. Continued research and coordinated professional training in diagnosis, treatment, and follow-up will be needed to unravel the tangled web and improve the quality and ultimate effectiveness of patient care.

References

Balter, M. B. An analysis of psychotherapeutic drug consumption in the United States. *Anglo-American Conference on Drug Abuse,* 1973, 1, 58-65.

Barchas, J. D., Berger, P. A., Ciaranell, R. D., & Elliot, G. R. (Eds.). *Psychopharmacology: From theory to practice.* New York: Oxford University Press, 1977.

Biegel, D., Naparstek, A., & Khan, M. Social support and mental health: An examination of interrelationships. Paper presented at the 88th Annual Meeting of the American Psychological Association, Montreal, September 1-5, 1980.

Brown, B. S., Regier, D. A., & Balter, M. B. Key interactions among psychiatric disorders, primary care and the use of psychotropic drugs. In B. S. Brown (Ed.), *Clinical anxiety-tension in primary medicine.* Princeton, NJ: Excerpta Medica, 1978.

Browning, D. H., Miller, S. I., & Tyson, R. L. The psychiatric emergency: A high risk medical patient. *Comprehensive Psychiatry,* 1974, 15, 153-159.

Burns, B. J., Orso, C., Jacobsen, A., Leet, R., & Goldner, N. Utilization of health and mental health outpatient services in organized medical care settings. Final report for NIMH Contract No. 278-76-10027. Baltimore, Maryland, 1977.

Cooper, C. C., & Payne, R. *Stress at work.* New York: John Wiley, 1978.

Davison, K., & Bagley, C. R. Schizophrenic-like psychoses associated with organic disorders of the central nervous system: A review of the literature. *British Journal of Psychiatry,* 1969, 4, 113-184.

Depue, R. A. *The psychobiology of depression.* New York: Academic Press, 1980.

Dohrenwend, B. P., & Dohrenwend, B. S. *Social status and psychological disorder.* New York: Wiley-Interscience, 1969.

Eastwood, M. R. *The relation between physical and mental illness.* Toronto: University of Toronto Press, 1975.

Eastwood, M. R., & Trevelyan, M. H. Relationship between physical and psychiatric disorder. *Psychological Medicine,* 1972, 2, 363-372.

Goldberg, D. P., & Blackwell, B. Psychiatric illness in general practice: A detailed study using a new method of case identification. *British Medical Journal,* 1970, 2, 439-443.

Goldberg, D. P., Cooper, B., Eastwood, M. R., Kedward, H. B., & Shepherd, M. A standardized psychiatric interview for use in community surveys. *British Journal of Preventive and Social Medicine,* 1970, 24, 18-23.

Goplerud, E. N. Unexpected consequences of deinstitutionalization of the mentally disabled elderly. *American Journal of Community Psychology,* 1979, 7, 315-328.

Goplerud, E. N. Social support and stress during the first year of graduate school. *Professional Psychology,* 1980, 33, 283-290.

Goplerud, E. N., Depue, R., Slater, J., & Fisher, A. Cyclothymia and dysthymia: A longitudinal investigation of characteristic behaviors of two high risk depressive groups. *Journal of
Abnormal Psychology,* in press.

Gori, G., & Richter, B. J. Macroeconomics of disease prevention in the United States. *Science,*
1978, 200, 1124-1130.

Hankin, J., & Oktay, J. S. *Mental disorder and primary medical care: An analytic review of the
literature.* DHEW Publication No. (ADM) 78-661. Washington, DC: Government Printing
Office, 1979.

Hänninen, H. Changes in performance, personality and subjective well-being as indicators of
long-term exposure to toxic environments. *Advances in Pharmacology and Therapeutics,*
1978, 9, 169-177.

Hoenig, J., & Hamilton, M. W. Mortality of psychiatric patients. *Acta Psychiatrica Scandinavica,* 1966, 42, 349-361.

Hoeper, E. W. Observations on the impact of psychiatric disorders upon primary medical care.
In D. L. Parron & F. Solomon (Eds.), *Mental health services in primary care settings.*
DHHS Publication No. (ADM) 80-995. Washington, DC: Government Printing Office,
1980.

Hoeper, E. W., Nycz, G. R., & Cleary, P. D. The quality of mental health services in an
organized primary health care setting. Final report to NIMH. Baltimore, Maryland, 1979.

Houpt, J. L., Orleans, C. S., George, L. K., & Brodie, H. K. H. *The importance of mental
health services to general health care.* Cambridge, MA: Ballinger, 1979.

Houpt, J. L., Orleans, C. S., George, L. K., & Brodie, H. K. H. The role of psychiatric and
behavioral factors in the practice of medicine. *American Journal of Psychiatry,* 1980, 137,
37-47.

Jacobs, T. L., Gogelson, S., & Charles, E. Depression ratings in hypochondria. *New York State
Journal of Medicine,* 1968, 68, 3119-3122.

Jacobson, A. M., Goldberg, I. D., Burns, B., Hoeper, E., Hankin, J. R., & Hewitt, K. Diagnosed mental disorders in children and use of health services in four organized health care
settings. *American Journal of Psychiatry,* 1980, 137, 559-565.

Jones, K. R., & Vischi, T. R. Impact of alcohol, drug abuse and mental health treatment on
medical care utilization: A review of the research literature. *Medical Care* (Supplement),
1979, 17.

Kampmeier, R. H. Diagnosis and treatment of physical diseases in the mentally ill. *Annals of
Internal Medicine,* 1977, 86, 637-645.

Kaplan, H. I., Freedman, A. M., & Sadock, B. J. *Comprehensive textbook of psychiatry/III.*
Baltimore, MD: Williams and Wilkins, 1980.

Kline, N. S., & Simpson, G. Lithium in the treatment of conditions other than affective
disorders. In S. Gershon & B. Simpsin (Eds.), *Lithium: Its role in psychiatric research and
treatment.* New York: Plenum, 1973.

Kolb, L. C., *Yearbook of psychiatry and applied mental health.* Chicago: Year Book Medical
Publishers, 1976.

Koranyi, E. K. Physical health and illness in a psychiatric outpatient department population.
Canadian Psychiatric Association Journal (Supplement), 1972, 17, 109-116.

Koranyi, E. K. Fatalities in 2070 psychiatric outpatients: Preventive features. *Archives of
General Psychiatry,* 1977, 34, 1137-1142.

Koranyi, E. K. Morbidity and rate of undiagnosed physical illnesses in a psychiatric clinic
population. *Archives of General Psychiatry,* 1979, 36, 414-419.

Leeman, C. P. Diagnostic errors in emergency room medicine: Physical illnesses in patients labeled "psychiatric" and vice versa. *International Journal of Psychiatric Medicine*, 1975, 6, 533-540.

Lipowski, Z. J. Psychiatry of somatic diseases: Epidemiology, pathogenesis, classification. *Comprehensive Psychiatry*, 1975, 16, 105-124.

McKegney, P. F. The incidence and prevalence of patients with conversion reactions: 1. A general hospital consultation service sample. *American Journal of Psychiatry*, 1967, 124, 542-547.

McLean, E. K., & Tarnopolsky, A. Noise discomfort and mental health: A review of the socio-medical implications of disturbance by noise. *Psychological Medicine*, 1977, 7, 19-62.

Maguire, G. P., & Granville-Grossman, K. L. Physical illness in psychiatric patients. *British Journal of Psychiatry*, 1968, 115, 1365-1371.

Martin, M. Psychiatry in medicine. In H. J. Kaplan, A. M. Freedman, & B. J. Sadock (Eds.), *Comprehensive textbook of psychiatary/III*. Baltimore, MD: Williams and Wilkins, 1980.

NIOSH (National Institute for Occupational Safety and Health). *Shift work and health: A symposium*. DHEW Publication No. (NIOSH) 76-203. Washington, DC: Government Printing Office, 1976.

Palarea, E. R. Medical evaluation of the psychiatric patient. *Journal of the American Geriatric Society*, 1965, 13, 14-19.

Rabkin, J. G. Stressful life events and schizophrenia: A review of the research literature. *Psychological Bulletin*, 1980, 87, 408-425.

Rabkin, J. G., & Struening, E. L. Life events, stress and illness. *Science*, 1976, 194, 1013-1020.

Regier, D. A. Nature and scope of mental health problems in primary care. In D. Parron & F. Solomon (Eds.), *Mental health services in primary care settings: Report of a conference April 2-3, 1979*. DHHS Publication No. (ADM) 80-995. Washington, DC: Government Printing Office, 1980.

Regier, D. A., Goldberg, I. D., & Taube, C. A. The de facto U.S. mental health services system. *Archives of General Psychiatry*, 1978, 35, 685-693.

Rorsman, B. Mortality among psychiatric patients. *Acta Psychiatrica Scandinavica*, 1974, 50, 354-375.

Rossman, P. L. Organic diseases resembling functional disorders. *Hospital Medicine*, 1969, 5, 72-76.

Schwab, J. J. Depression in medical and surgical patients. In A. J. Enlow (Ed.), *Depression in medical practice*. West Point, VA: Merck Sharp and Dohme, 1970.

Schwab, J. J., Bell, R. A., Warheit, G., & Schwab, R. B. *Social order and mental health*. New York: Brunner/Mazel, 1979.

Shader, R. I. (Ed.). *Psychiatric complications of medical drugs*. New York: Raven Press, 1972.

Shepherd, M., Cooper, B., Brown, A. C., & Kalton, G. W. *Psychiatric illness in general practice*. London: Oxford University Press, 1966.

U.S. DHEW (U.S. Department of Health, Education and Welfare). *Employees in nursing and personal care homes: U.S., May-June, 1964*. Publication No. 1000, Series 12(5). Washington, DC: Government Printing Office, 1966.

Waitzkin, L. A survey for unknown diabetes in a mental hospital: 1. Men under 50. *Diabetes*, 1966, 15, 97-104. (a)

Waitzkin, L. A survey for unknown diabetes in a mental hospital: 2. Men from age 50. *Diabetes,* 1966, 15, 164-172. (b)

Weiner, H. *Psychobiology and human disease.* New York: Elsevier, 1977.

Woodruff, R. A., Goodwin, D. W., & Guze, S. B. *Psychiatric diagnosis.* New York: Oxford University Press, 1974.

WHO (World Health Organization). Report on a working group convened by the Regional Office for Europe of the World Health Organization. Psychiatry and primary medical care. Lysebu, Oslo, April 10-13, 1973.

5

Alternative Funding and Incentive Mechanisms

Brian T. Yates
The American University

Nancy Marwick DeMuth
Johns Hopkins University

Current mental and physical health services are more costly than is necessary and less effective than is possible. Health service funding mechanisms, not health care providers, are at fault. The fiscal environment in which health services are delivered provides no systematic or concrete incentive for either maximizing effectiveness or minimizing cost. Government attempts to use regulations rather than rewards for effectiveness maximization and cost minimization have failed. For the health care provider, humanitarian desires to provide consumers with the most effective and least costly service are pitted against monetary incentives to provide as many consumers as possible with the most costly and lengthy treatment available. Practitioners are penalized for time spent measuring or attempting to improve their effectiveness or cost, because the same time could have been spent seeing more patients and making more money. The economic environment producing the high cost and questionable effectiveness of health services needs to be restructured: Providers must be rewarded for improving effectiveness and reducing cost.

This chapter first documents the present, growing cost of health services. Next, dilemmas posed by current health services funding mechanisms are analyzed. We show how attempts to improve effectiveness and reduce cost

Correspondence should be sent to Dr. Brian T. Yates, Department of Psychology, The American University, Nebraska and Massachusetts Avenues, N.W., Washington, D.C. 20016. Order of authors is arbitrary; both contributed equally to this chapter. During manuscript preparation the second author was supported as a postdoctoral research fellow by NIMH Grant No. 5T32MH14567-05.

by increased government regulation of the health industry have failed. Finally, three alternative ways for improving effectiveness and reducing cost in health services are suggested. We propose that a new funding environment replace the current cost-maximizing monopoly with nonmonopolistic incentives that reward the most effective and least costly providers. To answer criticisms of this proposal, and to detect and solve its problems in the present form, the recommended funding changes should be researched prior to implementation. Each of the three funding contingencies should be evaluated for effectiveness and cost-effectiveness after small-scale trials in representative communities. Rather than debate the possible positive and negative effects of the recommended funding revisions, we prefer to compare the actual effectiveness and cost of health services under the proposed versus the present funding system.

The Cost of Health Services

At present, physical and mental health services are a most costly and peculiar industry. Licensed providers in the United States have legal yet private monopolies on services required by every man, woman, and child some time during their lives. Because health service providers also discourage competition within their ranks, they have practically no financial incentive to improve or even monitor the effectiveness or cost of their services. Perhaps as a result, health services consumed a combined 11 percent of the Gross National Product in the mid-1970s (8 percent for physical and 3 percent for mental health services; see Yates, 1980a). Physical health services alone cost an average of $638 per U.S. citizen in 1975 (Gibson & Mueller, 1976). Physical health services promise to require 10 to 12 percent of the GNP by 1990 (Yates, 1980a). Thus, even if the mental health share of the GNP remains constant at 3 percent, a projected 13 to 15 percent of the 1990 GNP will be spent on mental and physical health services. The implication of these statistics is profound. Consider, for example, the expenditures of General Motors for employee health services. Private health insurers such as Blue Cross and Blue Shield are the largest single "supplier" to General Motors; Metropolitan Life Insurance is the second largest, U.S. Steel is a distant third (Zink, 1976).

If this was any other industry, health services would have been abandoned long ago by consumers. When the mental well-being, physical health, or very life of the consumer is at stake, however, it is difficult not to pay the price required. This is the central dilemma faced now by the consumer seeking health services: your money or your health? Government agencies, insurance corporations, employers, unions, and other "third parties" have taken the edge off difficult choices between money and health. Many consumers pay third parties in advance for physical and mental health services, filling the coffers and stock portfolios of third parties while removing the act of payment from the act of choosing a provider. As a result, the consumer has little incentive to seek the least costly provider. Because the consumer is not motivated to minimize health service costs, neither is the provider. Here, then, is a second dilemma spawned by the first. Other service industries minimize costs and maximize effectiveness under the threat of bankruptcy through consumer abandonment to competitors, but health services do not because there are no real competitors and because consumers are not motivated to minimize cost.

A third dilemma is created by the lack of information on the cost or effectiveness of alternative health service providers. Even if there were incentives for consumers to seek the least expensive and most beneficial provider, there are little data on which to base the sort of "comparison shopping" that keeps costs down and quality up in other industries. Although mental and physical health professions have been moved to allow advertising, little advertising has occurred. Even if costs were advertised, consumers might fear that the least expensive health service provider also would be the least effective. Because the effectiveness of different health service providers remains largely unadvertised and unmeasured, even consumers who wish to minimize the cost and maximize the effectiveness of health services cannot.

Costs of health services can be minimized and benefits of health services maximized only if all three dilemmas outlined are solved: (a) the private monopoly of health service providers, (b) the lack of consumer incentive to seek the least costly and most effective providers, and (c) the lack of information on the cost and effectiveness of alternative providers.

Dilemmas in Funding and Delivering Health Services

The public not only wants better physical and mental health services, but it wants them at lower cost (see Fielding, 1979; Weisbrod, Test, & Stein, 1980). These desires are thwarted by unique characteristics of the health industry, such as monopolistic privilege favoring one-provider dominance of all health services, and unintended but perverse effects of third-party funding mechanisms. Both characteristics are the result of earlier government efforts to improve health service effectiveness and reduce health service cost. Government granted physicians monopolies on physical and mental health services in the hope that the best training and most rigorous selection would assure the highest possible quality and effectiveness. Government later extended the monopoly for mental health services to psychologists, social workers, and psychiatric nurses. The result in both the mental and physical health arenas has been inflated prices and patched-on regulatory bodies impotent to either improve effectivenss or reduce cost.

When the monopoly held by psychologists, physicians, psychiatric nurses, and psychiatric social workers generated high costs, third parties such as insurance companies, unions, and the government stepped in to shift the burden from the consumer at one point in time (when health services are needed) to all potential consumers (all payers of premiums and taxes) over long periods of time (that is, over the wage-earning lifetime of each potential consumer). This appeared to benefit consumers by taking much of the pain out of paying for health services via reductions in immediate out-of-pocket expenditures. Government officials, citizens, and some health service professionals now question whether the benefits of these two prior "cures" for deleterious side effects of health service monopolies and increasing public funding of health services are worth the additional side effects (Magaro, Gripp, McDowell & Miller, 1978; Sharfstein, Towery, & Milowe, 1980). We detail these side effects in the following sections before turning to alternative "cures" that may be less iatrogenic.

Effects of Monopoly in Physical and Mental Health Services

Over a decade ago Bowen and Jeffers (1971) aptly summarized the negative effects of physician monopoly and public support of physical health services. The same analysis now fits the Ph.D.-M.D.-M.S.W.-R.N. monopoly on mental health services. Bowen and Jeffers (1971) describe a fragmented health industry in which there are no financial incentives for cost containment and no dissemination of consumer-oriented information about health service effectiveness and cost:

The bulk of the demand for services is mediated through physicians or is exercised collectively rather than by individuals. The industry tends to be highly inflexible; does not use resources efficiently; and is inequitable in terms of the health services made available to certain geographic areas, age groups, and income classes. The system is characterized by overuse and misuse of services; poor adjustments of the quantity of services supplied to changes in demand; and price escalation, as growth in insurance, income, and public expenditures give rise to increased outlays on health [p. 22].

Magaro et al. (1978) and O'Keefe and McCullough (1979) go farther, concluding that the health service industry is, like all monopolies,

- (1) one-producer dominated, with excessive provider power reinforced by state licensing laws, control of medical, clinical psychology, and other professional education, and control of third-party reimbursement strategies;

- (2) immune and unresponsive to supply-and-demand pressures due to its monopolistic rather than free market structure;

- (3) operating with prohibitive barriers to entry of competitors, as evidenced by exclusion of nonphysician providers from hospital privileges, exclusion of all but physicians from independent reimbursement under Medicaid and Medicare, and exclusion of any other than the four core mental health professions (M.D., Ph.D., R.N., M.S.W.) from practice in most areas; and

- (4) subject to producer rather than consumer control over prices and assessment of service quality.

Physicians and recognized mental health care providers are not solely or perhaps even primarily responsible for the present condition and expense of health services. Government and insurance companies have created the present health service system via their regulation and funding of it. Unions frequently demand "first-dollar" (no deductible) health coverage, all paid for by the employer. A major percentage of persons seeking and receiving physical and mental health services may be the "worried well" who consume practitioner time unnecessarily and drive up health services costs (Jones & Vischi, 1979). Questionable but expensive malpractice suits and inflation also are partly responsible for the dramatic rise in health service costs.

In sum, the cost and effectiveness of health services are functions of numerous factors. Suboptimal effectiveness and unnecessary cost are maintained by a complex of groups with a vested interest in maintaining the current funding system. Regrettably, most efforts to reduce costs and improve effectiveness have focused solely on the physician rather than on other providers or interest groups. Almost ignored have been the funding contingencies that are primarily responsible for less than optimally effective and overly expensive health services.

Attempts to Reduce Monopoly
in Health Services by Regulation

Federal moves to curb excessive power gained by physicians as a result of their federally endorsed monopoly inadvertently solidified that monopoly and power. No doubt similar moves are planned for recognized mental health providers such as psychologists. Similarly dismal results may be expected. Efforts to circumscribe physician power in health service delivery, such as establishment of professional standards review organizations (PSROs) and health systems agencies (HSAs), backfired. PSROs and HSAs created new areas in which physicians expressed their dominance (Stone, 1980). Legislation to enhance consumer representation on PSROs and HSAs, and to encourage innovative delivery systems such as health maintenance organizations (HMOs), also have failed to distribute power equitably (O'Keefe & McCullough, 1979; Starr, 1980). Antitrust actions by the Federal Trade Commission (FTC) to introduce free market competition in the health industry, to challenge single-provider control of private insurers such as Blue Shield, and to examine professional boycotts of HMOs, likewise had little impact (O'Keefe & McCullough, 1979; Starr, 1980).

Minor changes in health service provision resulted from government intervention but only chipped away at a massive problem. Under FTC pressure, the American Medical Association endorsed advertising by physicians. Should advertising of health service costs become widespread, prices may become lower as they did in optometry once advertising was allowed (Bloom & Stiff, 1980). Court actions produced consumer "freedom of choice" statutes in 29 states and the District of Columbia (Professionally Speaking, 1980) that require insurance corporations to directly reimburse mental health services provided by recognized nonphysician providers (American Psychological Association, 1979). Major changes in physician dominance of physical health services seem unlikely, however. As nonphysician providers such as psychologists, psychiatric social workers, and psychiatric nurses gain an independent slice of the health care dollar, they too will find it profitable to resist further demonopolization that would allow additional competition.

Effects of Attempts to Reduce
Health Service Costs

Efforts to reduce the cost of health services through insurance and regulation have been largely unsuccessful and have themselves added to the total health services bill. Private health insurance does not reduce the actual cost of health services but simply spreads health service costs over a longer period of time and among all premium payers. The primary benefits of health insurance are more equitable distribution of catastrophic health service costs and increased funds available for investment in other industries. The costs of health insurance are many. The cost of operating insurance corporations is added to the basic cost of health services. Health insurance also may increase health service costs by removing consumer incentives to shop for the least expensive provider, thus removing provider incentives to minimize cost themselves. A disincentive for hiring workers is provided by several states' requirement that employers purchase health insurance for employees.

Now paying for over 30 percent of all health services (White, 1979), Medicaid and Medicare are similar to private insurance, except that their costs are distributed involuntarily over an even broader population—all taxpayers. Medicaid and Medicare also motivate excessive health costs. Overcharging by providers is well documented and may be complied with by consumers who do not directly pay the extra price. Overcharging Medicare and Medicaid also can benefit local economies by drawing in outside tax monies (McClue, 1978). Overuse of medications paid for by public health insurance is common and can be stopped only if expensive computer networks link different pharmacies into a common memory of drug prescriptions filled (Medical World News, 1980). In their present form, Medicaid and Medicare also reimburse easily monitored inpatient treatment more readily than day- or outpatient treatment, even though day- and outpatient treatment are at least as effective and considerably less expensive (Penk, Charles & Vanhoose, 1978; Weisbrod et al., 1980).

Regulations attempting to improve effectiveness of publicly funded health services failed, just as they failed for privately funded services. Amendments passed in 1972 to improve service quality for Medicaid and Medicare patients via PSROs required expenditures of so much money that their effects were judged not worth the cost by government evaluations. Attempts to regulate health insurance through claims review generated inaccurate data on client dysfunctions and sabotaged meaningful peer review of health service effectiveness (Sharfstein et al., 1980). Government-funded alternatives to private mental health care and public mental hospitals did not succeed and slowly are being abandoned. For example, at least some community mental health centers (usually private health services receiving public funding) provided ineffective services to deinstitutionalized mental patients and criminals needing rehabilitation (Dorken, 1980). Funding for CMHCs is being reduced, and the broad range of services previously mandated are no longer required.

Private industry should be in the forefront of health service cost reduction, because it bears a major proportion of health care expenses and because
its profits are affected by the cost and effectiveness of health services. Health
benefits also are a major cause of management-worker disagreements and
ensuing shutdowns. Health benefit issues generated the longest strikes in the
1970s at both Ford Motor Corporation and General Motors. Only preliminary efforts have been made by private industry to revise health services (see
Chapter 8 by Manuso). The results are promising but inadequate as yet.
General Motors asks for second opinions about the necessity of surgery.
Kennecott Copper and other firms have been subsidizing psychotherapy for
drug abuse and other mental health problems because psychotherapy seems
more cost-beneficial than remedial physical health services (see Cummings
& Follette, 1968, 1976; Kennecott Copper Corporation, 1975).

Unfortunately, these changes work within the existing monopolistic and
insurance-dominated health services system. A more radical and different
course is suggested by the failure of repeated attempts to change the current
system. New strategies are needed that are more than bandages on fatal
flaws in the present health services delivery system. Moreover, because
prior attempts to reduce cost and improve effectiveness in health services
have failed, these new strategies need to be tested in small-scale implemen-
tations before widespread adoption.

Toward Self-Optimizing and Self-Correcting Systems for Delivering Physical and Mental Health Services

Reimbursement Based on Effectiveness and Cost, Not Just Process

The ways in which physical and mental health services now are reimbursed by consumers and insurers reinforces providers for executing accepted treatment processes but ignores the effectiveness of those processes
and their cost. We doubt that these funding procedures were designed to
avoid accountability to consumers and funders. When current funding
mechanisms were designed, the effectiveness of health services either was
assumed (e.g., tonsillectomy, radical mastectomy) or seemed impossible or
irrelevant to measure (e.g., psychoanalysis, treatment of the terminally ill).
Funders could only ask practitioners to keep fees, tests, and equipment
charges within reason. The actual process of delivering health services was
assumed to be the best possible because the practitioner held an advanced

degree and was licensed. If actions of the client prevented processes from being properly executed (e.g., nonadherence to self-medication, skipping therapy appointments), it was the patient's fault.

All this has changed in the last decade. The acceptance and growth of research in all health service areas, from surgery to psychotherapy, has forced empirical examination of "standard" procedures that were once assumed effective. Some of these were found to be no more effective than no or placebo treatments (see Garfield & Bergin, 1978). Health scientists now quantify the effectiveness of different treatments with multiple measures that have been validated in previous studies (see Kazdin, 1980). Some health researchers also now quantify the costs of different treatments with multiple measures such as time and income foregone by clients during treatment, psychological suffering endured by clients and family, and the actual as well as the reported amount of practitioner time and other resources consumed during treatment (e.g., Yates, 1980b). The cost-benefit and cost-effectiveness of different medical and mental regimens (such as annual gynecological tests, regular chest x-rays, psychotherapy) not only are being computed but also are beginning to determine whether the regimens are or are not funded by health insurance (e.g., Yates, 1980a; Yates & Newman, 1980a, 1980b).

Evaluators of health services do not assume that health care techniques have been competently implemented. "Internal evaluations" are conducted routinely to check on the thoroughness with which service processes were implemented. The patient no longer is the only one blamed if he or she does not adhere to a regimen. Development and testing of procedures for maximizing client adherence to and participation in treatment are beginning (e.g., Danaher & Lichtenstein, 1978; Zifferblatt, 1975). These advances in effectiveness and cost measurement, and these changes in the way in which practitioner and client roles are viewed, now allow funding of health services to be based on the worth of the product and the cost of obtaining it as well as on the processes used to deliver it.

The primary question faced by funders of health services, from insurance agencies to private individuals, is exactly how to link reimbursement for health services to effectiveness, adequacy of implementation, and cost of the consumer and taxpayers. Optimally this "linkage" would require minimal government regulation and would need little adjustment when new health care technologies or demands were introduced. For mental health services, pending federal legislation would establish a board comprised of recognized care providers to determine which treatment techniques are or are not effective according to research and to sponsor further research. This is a laudable step in the right direction, but it may not go far enough and may again amount to only more regulation of the health industry. The legislation assumes that mental health services are analogous to drugs and can be standardized and tested in the same manner. The legislation assumes that findings can be generalized to all providers and ignores the cost-effectiveness and cost-benefit of different services. The effectiveness, cost-effectiveness, and cost-benefit of mental and physical health services may be more a function of the provider than the technique, and certainly involve an interaction of the two (Garfield & Bergin, 1978).

Rather than mandate by legislation only one of many possible revisions of health services funding, we believe that alternative funding strategies for linking effectiveness and cost-effectiveness to provider reimbursement should be tested by actual trial implementation in a variety of communities. The effectiveness and cost-effectiveness of each revision should then be measured and the optimal revision implemented, perhaps in different forms that are best suited to different communities according to data collected in the trial studies. Possible forms of effectiveness- and cost-linked funding systems are explored below.

Alternatives for Building Incentives into Health Services Funding

There are literally thousands of ways in which effectiveness and cost could be linked to provider reimbursement. Any of three interest groups could introduce effectiveness maximization and cost minimization incentives into health services funding: (1) consumers, (2) third-party funders, and (3) providers. There are seven possible alliances of these interest groups that might influence the success of incentives offered. To assess the degree to which different practitioner-consumer combinations attain the effectiveness maximation within constraints goal, and to use the assessment in funding decision rules, effectiveness and cost need to be defined operationally and data collected on each. The four principal sources of definitions and data for the effectiveness and costs of health services are (a) consumers and those interacting with consumers (e.g., family, employers), (b) third-party funders, (c) service providers, and (d) independent testing or evaluation firms. There are 14 possible combinations of these. The number of alternative funding systems is already $7 \times 14 = 98$. Multiply this by the number of alternative time periods over which effectiveness and cost measures could be collected before being fed into the reimbursement decision process (e.g., a year, the end of service for a given client), and the specific decision rules that might be employed (e.g., reimburse a fixed amount with extra reimbursement for superior effectiveness or lower-than-average charges), and the alternatives for funding health services become too numerous to consider all of them here.

We will concentrate on some of the more promising and general funding systems. Different approaches to assessing effectiveness need not be considered at this point. Much research has shown that the effectiveness, benefits, costs, cost-effectiveness, and cost-benefit of physical and mental health services can be measured with reasonable accuracy using a variety of measures (see Thompson, 1980; Yates, 1980b; Yates & Newman, 1980a, 1980b). Measures appropriate for one type of health service will not be appropriate for others and will have to be tailored to the dysfunction treated. Also, the time period over which effectiveness and cost data are collected before making reimbursement decisions probably will be determined largely by the decision makers (those controlling funding) and by the particular decision rules used. This simplifies the number of alternatives to be investigated. Below we outline three major approaches that seem worth implementing on a trial basis for statistical comparison against each other and against current health service funding schemes.

Funding Scenario #1
Third Parties Determine Reimbursement, One-Year Time Frame,
Decision Rule: Deviation from Average Effectiveness or Cost

If third parties such as government agencies or private insurance firms are the primary decision makers in health services funding, it seems best to reimburse providers according to their past deviation from the average effectiveness or cost for practitioners in the locale treating similar dysfunctions (see Magaro et al., 1978). In this centralized funding scenario to be researched, a time period of a year for data collection might be optimal after operational definitions of service effectiveness, process, and cost have been agreed upon. One year should allow ample time for surveys of clients, therapists, and others to collect effectiveness and cost data. Less than a year may be required if the primary data collectors and analyzers are private testing firms that can be expected to be more responsive to time constraints. Effectiveness, process, and cost data for each provider or service agency would be reported to the third-party funder. To minimize costs and maximize adequacy of the data collected, different firms could bid for the data collector/analyst contract each year, as is common in other human services evaluation (such as Head Start).

Deviation from the mean effectiveness index used seems a fair basis for reimbursement decisions. There would, however, be much argument over what constituted a deviation and how much was significant enough to affect the amount reimbursed. The safest decision rule might be to assume a normal distribution of effectiveness (as found for mental health services by Smith, Glass, & Miller, 1980), and to reimburse the standard fee set by current procedures for providers generating effectiveness indices within a half standard deviation on either side of mean effectiveness. This would, by definition of the normal distribution, give more than a third of all providers the standard fee. Providers exceeding a one-half standard deviation might receive additional reimbursement proportional to the percentage of the local effectiveness distribution at which their mean effectiveness was located. For example, if a practitioner produced services of an average effectiveness 1.0 standard deviation above the mean effectiveness for the locale and dysfunction, their effectiveness is at about the 84th percentile of the normal distribution and they should receive payment of 100% + 84% = 184% of the standard fee. A practitioner with an average effectiveness 1.0 standard deviation below the mean would be at roughly the 16th percentile and would receive 16% of the standard or requested fee. The exact number or fraction of a standard deviation used as the cutoff for standard reimbursement could be researched for maximal effectiveness and minimal disruption of the health services system.

Overall, there would be practically no change in the total reimbursement paid by the funder if the above decision rule used the standard fee awarded previously without reference to effectiveness. The above decision rule is fixed to the mean: The extra money paid to the more effective practitioner would be the money not paid to the less effective practitioner. As the overall effectiveness of health services improved, the total amount of money paid to practitioners would remain almost the same unless the number of practitioners entering the market exceeded the number leaving due to loss of income and retirement. The prediction of no change in funding also assumes maintenance of the normal distribution of effectiveness scores for different providers after the funding contingency has been put in place. If the distribution changed from normal to Poisson or another skewed distribution, the same percentage-based decision rule could be applied as long as standard deviation was calculated according to the formula appropriate for the distribution obtained. There would be a moderate increase in costs for the collection, analysis, and dissemination of cost and effectiveness data. The question to be answered by research on the proposed funding strategy is whether this addition cost is worth the increased effectiveness of health services produced.

Implementation of this "from those who are less effective to those who are more effective" funding mechanism could have positive effects aside from rewarding superior effectiveness and low cost. It might compel providers to seek and reimburse the services of consultant research firms that would work with providers to improve effectiveness and reduce cost, based perhaps on cost, process, and effectiveness data collected internally by the consultants (see Yates, 1980b). Implementation of the proposed funding decision scheme also would provide incentives for physicians and others to encourage entry of other providers into the industry. If these providers are less effective, as they are alleged to be, then physicians, clinical psychologists, and other recognized providers have much to gain by allowing others to enhance the lower end and middle of the effectiveness distribution. Thus, all three of the dilemmas noted earlier as created by the present funding system could be mitigated by this revision of health services funding.

New techniques or practitioners who met new demands also would be amply rewarded with increased income for their superior effectiveness. Innovators might be allowed a period of unconditional funding to allow the adjustments in treatment process integral to research and development of new techniques. Innovators would be required, however, eventually to publish findings of experiments comparing the cost and effectiveness of their services to others. Care would have to be taken in the definition of "innovation" lest all service providers argue that health services are by their very nature continual innovation.

Naturally, many other decision rules could be applied if funding is controlled centrally by third parties. Regardless of the specific rule used, it would be important to collect effectiveness data on a continuing basis to allow practitioners who improved in effectiveness to be rewarded for that and to maintain the effectiveness of other practitioners. Use of a shorter time period for data collection and revision of reimbursement rates for individual providers should automatically increase the rate of service improvement.

Application of similar funding decision rules to cost minimization as well as effectiveness maximization seems more complex but necessary. If some cost-linkage is not made, however, and if practitioners are allowed to set their own fees, charges would no doubt be raised by the practitioner if effectiveness was anticipated to be low. This would defeat the cost stabilization factor built into the "deviation" decision rule. A standard "base" fee for each service could be set, from which an amount was subtracted or added according to the standard deviations from the effectiveness mean. Alternatively, the standard deviation decision rule might be applied independently to the fee requested by the practitioner. In this case, the fee request would be treated just as effectiveness data were, with reimbursement set inversely proportional to the percentage of the fee distribution at which the requested fee fell. The results of this rule are difficult to anticipate, however. Practitioners presumably would set fees below the mean of all requested fees to reap additional reimbursement. All practitioners would make similar adjustments, however, and use of the compared-to-the-mean decision rule for reimbursement of lower- or higher-than-average costs still would provide an incentive to minimize costs. Costs may, of course, be better determined by a free market, as in the following scenario.

There are a number of problems to be worked out before this funding contingency could be implemented. Questions that come immediately to mind are:

(1) Who would pay for the effectiveness surveys?

(2) What effectiveness measures would be used?

(3) What prevents reporting of false, high effectiveness?

(4) Would the costs of administrating this contingency surpass its benefits in improved health care and reduced fees?

(5) How does this improve on the "reasonable and customary" reimbursement strategy now in place with Blue Cross and Blue Shield coverage?

Tentative answers come to mind, although they would have to be confirmed in research on pilot versions of the proposed contingency. Collection of effectiveness and cost data perhaps could be paid for through current health care funds by allowing practitioners to charge for time spent in data collection. Health service funders also could reimburse independent data collection agencies. The effectiveness measures used would be specific to the problems of the client, of course, but could be standardized just as mental dysfunctions have been standardized by the DSM-III and just as mental health treatments are being standardized by the PTM-I (Psychiatric Treatment Manual I). Practitioners would have incentives to try a variety of measures until they found one sensitive to their treatment effects.

Falsification of effectiveness data could be minimized by using independent data collection firms that obtain effectiveness data from the family and employer of patients as well as from the practitioner and patient themselves. The cost of data collection, analysis, and dissemination required by this first proposal could vary greatly depending on the measures used and frequency of data collection. Minimizing this cost and maximizing the effectiveness increment and cost decrement produced by the new funding contingency would be the job of pilot research. Finally, this and the following funding contingencies certainly are a change from the current system. The amount of reimbursement no longer is set by the practitioner irrespective of effectiveness and rejected if it is above the limit set by health care funders. Instead, reimbursement is set according to the effectiveness, and perhaps the cost, of the treatment provided.

Funding Scenario #2
Consumers and Their Representatives Determine Reimbursement,
Quarterly to Annual Time Frame, Decision Rule: Consumer Freedom of Choice

The first scenario keeps third parties in the driver's seat of health services funding. It allows health professionals to continue their control of funding levels and effectiveness criteria through lobbying insurance corporations and government. A more radical funding structure to be researched would give consumers the primary power to determine reimbursement by simply allowing it to function as a free enterprise (Buck & Hirschman, 1980; Magaro et al., 1978). Poor clients would be given health service vouchers, as has been proposed for educational services. If national health insurance was enacted, all consumers would receive vouchers. Consumers would peruse effectiveness and cost information made available for all potential health service providers. If the consumer was too disturbed or uneducated to make a rational, informed decision, representatives could be elected to "shop" for the consumer.

Effectiveness, process, and cost data on alternative providers could be collected, analyzed, and disseminated to consumers by contracted testing firms, as in Scenario #1. These data also could be collected, analyzed, and published by private firms, much as *Consumer Reports* now collects data on the performance of material goods. A healthy variety of data collection, analysis, and dissemination firms would arise if clients were allowed to spend part of their voucher to obtain effectiveness and cost information. Competition among firms that collect, analyze, and disseminate findings could be relied on to keep firms out of the control of providers and eventually to generate evaluations of the evaluation firms themselves. Health service organizations such as HMOs also might be expected to conduct their own effectiveness and cost assessments and to advertise the findings, just as automobile manufacturers and others do now with consumer preference surveys. There also would be an even greater incentive for health providers to seek services of research consultants so that the cost and effectiveness data collected could be used to improve, rather than simply assess, the health services provided (Yates, 1979).

As in other free enterprise sectors of the economy, consumers or their representatives would seek out and deliver the most profits to health practitioners who demonstrated superior quality of service and effective outcomes. As proposed by Long (1974), firms analogous to the American Automobile Association might evolve both to provide insurance and to make referrals to health service providers who meet set standards for effectiveness and cost. AAA-model health organizations could conduct the hard-nosed inspection of effectiveness, process, and cost statistics, publishing lists of the most effective and cost-effective providers.

Incentives for choosing providers who also minimize cost would be present for the individual consumer if the consumer paid directly for health services, but would have to be created if vouchers were used. Fortunately, a means for inducing consumers to minimize health service costs reimbursed by third parties already has been developed. The California Mendocino County Office of Education pays employees a percentage of the difference between the total health service payment available for the year and the amount actually spent by the client. The reduction produced in health service expenses was sufficient to prevent what had been a routine annual increase in health insurance premiums, even though the percentage reimbursed to employees was paid only when they terminated employment. More frequent reimbursement should produce even greater reduction in health service expenses. The proposed funding strategy would provide consumers with generous vouchers to pay well for effective services. Regular "rebate" of a percentage of unspent vouchers would encourage consumer shopping for less expensive providers and prevent unnecessary use of mental and physical health services. The exact voucher ceiling, percentage of unspent monies rebated, and time between voucher award and rebate could be adjusted via research to maximize incentives and minimize undue costs.

A variety of criticisms can be leveled at this second funding scenario, and certainly not all can be rebuted in this space. The strongest criticism would be doubt in the ability of individual consumers to shop intelligently for health services, the processes and results of which may require technical sophistication beyond the reach of most consumers. First, the ability of consumers may be underestimated by these critics. The small-scale experimental trial proposed earlier for each of the funding scenarios could collect information on consumer decisions and determine just how wise the consumer is. Second, should most consumers be shown to not have the requisite background for health services shopping, AAA-model firms as described above might provide the pooling of expertise needed to make intelligent health service decisions.

Funding Scenario #3
Practitioner and Third-Party Control of Reimbursement,
Consumer as Preventative Practitioner, Decision Rule:
Reimbursement Contingent on Low Health-Risk Behavior

The present health funding system and the two proposed above provide monies to consumers only when they are ineffective in efforts to prevent health problems, inadvertently reinforcing poor health maintenance. Some HMOs attempt to focus more on prevention than treatment. Many, however, are simply large insurance-based treatment clinics. An alternative is for third parties and others who control health services funding to monetarily reimburse the consumer and professionals for avoiding treatment by effectively self-managing health-related behaviors.

Consumers have in their hands a prime means of improving the effectiveness and reducing costs of health services: self-management of health-related behavior so that behaviors benefiting health are maximized and risk-taking behaviors are minimized. The physical and mental dysfunctions treated most commonly today are largely the result of past misbehavior of the consumer (Ferguson & Taylor, 1980). Cardiovascular dysfunction, character disorders, alcohol abuse, and other problems may be prevented not by the ministrations of professionals but by the potential consumers themselves. Proper diet, cessation of smoking, regular aerobic activity, minimization of overly stressful work, and the presence of social relationships seem closely related to a lower need for physical and mental health services. Such factors are controllable largely by the consumer. Moreover, prevention of a dysfunction may well be less costly in time, effort, and funds than treatment of a dysfunction. Finally, prevention of physical and mental health risk factors may make treatment of dysfunctions that do develop more successful (for example, lower mortality rates of corrective surgery for myocardioinfarctions in nonsmokers).

The consumer could be the front-line health practitioner. Consumers need incentives to avoid behaviors that are immediately pleasurable but that pose long-term health risks. If the consumer is successful in reducing health risks, he deserves to be rewarded for it. Psychologists and other practitioners of behavioral medicine can help consumers in self-management of health behaviors, as detailed in other chapters of this monograph (see also Cummings & Follette, 1968, 1976; Ferguson & Taylor, 1980). These practitioners also deserve funding proportional to their effectiveness in helping the consumer reduce health risks and thus save the consumer and funders money. Either of the above decision rules could be used to reimburse practitioners and consumers for prevention of high-risk behaviors.

A prevention-oriented incentive system for funding consumer-controlled health behaviors deserves to be included in research trials of alternative health services funding structures. Behaviors high in risk to physical or mental behavior can be identified from the large epidemiological literature now available (for example, Yates, 1980a). Potential consumers of health services would simply be paid to minimize occurrence of those behaviors. Except for problems of verifying consumer reports of risk-taking behavior, which can be solved largely by occasional chemical tests (such as long-lasting smoking byproducts in urine), paying consumers to stay healthy may well be less costly to health services funders than paying for professional services once consumers develop dysfunctions. The size of the monetary incentive offered for consumer reduction of health risk behavior would be set so that it was less than the probabilistic cost of treating the avoided dysfunctions but sufficient to motivate change in consumer behavior. Additional contingencies would have to be created to avoid making it profitable for consumers to first increase and then decrease health risk behaviors.

Some life insurance companies already have implemented consumer incentives for healthy behavior by offering lower rates to nonsmokers and teetotalers. Health insurance companies can do the same. Private funders of health services also have begun researching this preventive, behavioral medicine approach to revising health services funding. Some private industries seem already to have found that funding consumer efforts to avoid health risk behaviors are cost-beneficial. A few corporations now pay workers to self-manage their health so that use of treatment services will not be as necessary. For example, Sears, Roebuck, and Company of New York City rebates employees' tuition for smoking cessation programs if they stop smoking for at least 6 months. Other companies have paid bonuses to clients who maintain smoking cessation or who keep off excess weight for a year or more. Fielding (1979) reports that Mobil Corporation has used a more general form of health maintenance contingency for consumers. Mobil gives an annual bonus to employees who have stayed healthy and used less than the average medical coverage. Total bonuses distributed were $1.4 million in 1977 to 25,600 employees at a mean $55 per employee. Fielding also reports several insurance companies that provide lower premiums for persons minimizing health risk behaviors. It would be interesting indeed to compare the cost-effectiveness and cost-benefit of funding consumer-practitioner efforts to maintain and enhance physical and mental health to the previously described means of funding practitioners to mitigate physical and mental dysfunction.

Directions for Research

In summary, we argue that current funding mechanisms for health services are the result of preliminary and unsuccessful attempts to assure effective, high-quality health services by allowing only highly trained professionals to deliver health services. This effort created a monopoly on health care that has been immune to regulation by the federal government. Maintenance of present health funding is fostered by those who benefit from restrictions on practitioner recognition, by unions which demand the highest health insurance coverage available, by insurance firms which control the system by funding it, and by consumers who abuse health insurance by overuse and excessive malpractice litigation. The effectiveness maximization and cost minimization forces normally present in free market economies are largely absent in the health service monopoly. Under the funding contingency now in place, health providers are reimbursed for using standard treatment techniques and minimizing time spent per consumer as long as other consumers are available for servicing. Practitioners are "fined" if they take the time to measure, research, and thereby improve their effectiveness or cost. They also are unprepared for assessing and improving cost-effectiveness, due to the nature of most professional training.

Three basic strategies for introducing effectiveness maximization and cost minimization forces into the health services sector are proposed. Techniques for assessing and improving the effectiveness and cost-effectiveness of physical and mental health services have been developed and tested (see Yates, 1980a; Yates & Newman, 1980a, 1980b). These techniques allow linkage of practitioner reimbursement to demonstrated effectiveness and low cost, rather than solely to the professional degree obtained in graduate school.

In the first strategy, third-party funders collect data on the effectiveness and cost of each practitioner and reimburse practitioners according to their effectiveness and cost relative to other practitioners working with similar health problems. This "standard deviation" decision rule would not increase health costs appreciably but ideally would take funds from the less effective provider and give those funds to the more effective provider. A similar decision rule might be used to cut costs.

The second funding scenario would create a real rather than an artificial free enterprise system for health services funding. Third parties would simply provide vouchers to consumers. Practitioner licensing could be relaxed. Consumers would shop for the most effective and convenient health service. Consumers would also be motivated to minimize the cost of the health service chosen, as the consumer would receive a partial rebate of unused vouchers. Consumers also could spend part of their voucher to obtain information about the effectiveness and cost of alternative service providers. Publications analogous to *Consumer Reports* should emerge to assess, analyze, and report in easily grasped statistics the effectiveness and costs of alternative providers. Organizations similar to the American Automobile Association in the commercial sector might evolve to interpret effectiveness and cost data and to refer consumer members to effective and inexpensive practitioners.

The third funding scenario is compatible with either of the first two schemes, but provides consumer and practitioner incentives for prevention rather than just treatment of health problems. Consumers who demonstrate a reduction in health risk behaviors, or who maintain low levels of health risks, would be reimbursed, as would professionals who successfully assist consumers in self-management of health risk behaviors.

The above strategies, of course, are not guaranteed to work in their present form. All the effects of implementing them cannot be anticipated, and some of these effects undoubtedly will be negative. The above funding proposals have little hope of being installed at present; they should not be. We have outlined only the barest skeletons of only a few alternative funding strategies for health services. Much planning is needed to add substance to what we have sketched so simplistically. To identify the problems, to develop concrete and feasible funding arrangements, to select the most cost-effective funding strategy, and to motivate those in control of health funding to adopt new funding mechanisms, the above strategies need to be implemented on a small-scale trial basis.

First, the above strategies should be implemented in a small but representative sample of communities. The effectiveness and cost of health services under the new funding strategies could be assessed comprehensively over several years. Next, these data should be compared with both the prior effectiveness and cost of health services in the same communities and the effectiveness and cost of health services funded in the traditional manner in comparable communities during the same years. If none of the proposed funding innovations significantly and substantially improve effectiveness or reduce cost, the innovations should be discarded. If, however, there are notable improvements, a progressively larger scale of funding strategy implementation would ensue along with continued assessment and research.

Funding for the proposed research could be obtained from the federal government's health agencies and from third-party funders dissatisfied with current funding mechanisms. If the new funding strategies prove themselves worthwhile, adoption could be mandated by the federal government in concert with interested insurance and health maintenance organizations. Alternatively, lobbying and funding for the proposed research may come from private industries that bear an increasing burden of costs for current health services but that also control, via their premiums, an increasing portion of the health service industry. Private industry has been at the forefront of health service innovation, as examples in this chapter have illustrated. Given the high cost and questionable effectiveness of current health services caused largely by current funding mechanisms, private industry is likely to find any change in funding strategies to be cost-beneficial and may decide to fund the proposed research itself.

References

American Psychological Association. Information packet, Committee on Health Insurance. Washington, D.C., 1979.

Bloom, P. N., & Stiff, R. Advertising and health care professions. *Journal of Health Politics, Policy and Law,* 1980, 4, 642-656.

Bowen, H. R., & Jeffers, J. R. The economics of health services. New York: General Learning Press, 1971.

Buck, J. A., & Hirschman, R. Economics and mental health services. *American Psychologist,* 1980, 35, 653-661.

Cummings, N. A., & Follette, W. T. Psychiatric services and medical utilization in a prepaid health plan setting. *Medical Care,* 1968, 5, 31-41.

Cummings, N. A., & Follette, W. T. Brief psychotherapy and medical utilization: An eight-year follow-up. In H. Dorken et al. (Eds.), *The professional psychologist today: New developments in law, health insurance, and health practice.* San Francisco: Jossey-Bass, 1976.

Danaher, B. G., & Lichtenstein, E. *Become an ex-smoker.* Englewood Cliffs, NJ: Prentice-Hall, 1978.

Dorken, H. National health insurance: Implications for mental health practitioners. *Professional Psychology,* 1980, 11, 664-671.

Ferguson, J., & Taylor, C. B. (Eds.). *The comprehensive handbook of behavioral medicine, vol. 3.* Jamaica, NY: S & P Medical and Scientific, 1980.

Fielding, J. W. Preventative medicine and the bottom line. *Journal of Occupational Medicine,* 1979, 21, 79-88.

Garfield, S. L., & Bergin, A. E. (Eds.). *Handbook of psychotherapy.* New York: John Wiley, 1978.

Gibson, R. M., & Mueller, M. S. Research and statistics note 27. Bethesda, MD: National Institutes of Health, December 1976.

Jones, K. R., & Vischi, T. R. Impact of alcohol, drug abuse, and mental health treatment on medical care utilization: A review of the research literature. *Medical Care* (Supplement), 1979, 17.

Kazdin, A. E. *Research in clinical psychology.* New York: Holt, Rinehart & Winston, 1980.

Kennecott Copper Corporation. *Insight: A program for troubled people.* Salt Lake City: Utah Copper Division, 1975.

Long, N. A. A model for coordinating human services. *Administration in Mental Health,* 1974, Summer, 21-27.

McClure, W. An incentive tax for Medicare and national health insurance. *Journal of Health Politics, Policy and Law,* 1978, 5, 10-24.

Magaro, P. A., Gripp, R., McDowell, D. J., & Miller, I. W. *The mental health industry: A cultural phenomenon.* New York: John Wiley, 1978.

Medical World News. Computerizing cuts prescribing of psychotropics. September 4, 1980, 11-12.

O'Keefe, A. M., & McCullough, S. J. Physician domination in the health care industry: The pursuit of antitrust redress. *Professional Psychology,* 1979, 10, 605-618.

Penk, W. E., Charles, H. L., & Vanhoose, T. A. Comparative effectiveness of day hospital and inpatient psychiatric treatment. *Journal of Consulting and Clinical Psychology,* 1978, 46, 94-101.

Professionally Speaking. Memo from the American Psychological Assocation Office of Professional Affairs, No. 37, p. 1.

Sharfstein, S. S., Towery, O. B., & Milowe, I. D. Accuracy of diagnostic information submitted to an insurance company. *American Journal of Psychiatry,* 1980, 137, 70-73.

Smith, M. L., Glass, G. V., & Miller, T. I. *The benefits of psychotherapy.* Baltimore, MD: Johns Hopkins University Press, 1980.

Starr, P. Changing the balance of power in American medicine. *Milbank Memorial Fund Quarterly,* 1980, 58, 166-172.

Stone, D. A. The problem of monopoly power in federal health policy. *Milbank Memorial Fund Quarterly,* 1980, 58, 50-53.

Thompson, M. S. *Benefit-cost analysis for program evaluation.* Beverly Hills, CA: Sage, 1980.

Weisbrod, B. A., Test, M. A., & Stein, L. I. Alternatives to mental hospital treatment II: Economic benefit-cost analysis. *Archives of General Psychiatry,* 1980, 37, 400-405.

White, D. W. Why is regulation introduced in the health sector? A look at occupational licensure. *Journal of Health Politics, Policy and Law,* 1979, 4, 536-552.

Yates, B. T. How to improve, rather than evaluate, cost-effectiveness. *Counseling Psychologist,* 1979, 8, 72-75.

Yates, B. T. The theory and practice of cost-utility, cost-effectiveness, and cost-benefit analysis in behavioral medicine: Toward delivering more health care for less money. In J. Ferguson and C. B. Taylor (Eds.), *The comprehensive handbook of behavioral medicine, vol. 3.* Jamaica, NY: S & P Medical and Scientific, 1980. (a)

Yates, B. T. *Improving effectiveness and reducing costs in mental health.* Springfield, IL: Charles C Thomas, 1980. (b)

Yates, B. T., & Newman, F. L. Approaches to cost-effectiveness and cost-benefit analysis of psychotherapy. In G. VandenBos (Ed.), *Psychotherapy: From practice to research to policy.* Beverly Hills, CA: Sage, 1980. (a)

Yates, B. T., & Newman, F. L. Findings of cost-effectiveness and cost-benefit analyses of psychotherapy. In G. VandenBos (Ed.), *Psychotherapy: From practice to research to policy.* Beverly Hills, CA: Sage, 1980. (b)

Zifferblatt, S. M. Increasing patient compliance through the applied analysis of behavior. *Preventative Medicine,* 1975, 4, 173-182.

Zink, V. M. Testimony to Senator Kennedy's Subcommittee on Health. Washington, DC: Government Printing Office, 1976.

PART II

SERVICE DELIVERY MODELS

6

Mental Health Services in the Health Maintenance Organization

Simon H. Budman

*Harvard Community Health Plan,
Boston, Massachusetts*

This country is faced with a health care crisis of major proportions. The rising cost of receiving health care services is rapidly outstripping our current double-digit inflation and there is little reason to expect any relief in the near future.

Approximately 10 years ago, the Nixon administration, searching for a strategy to deal with rapidly rising medical care expenditures, chose to encourage the concept of health maintenance organizations (HMOs) as a central feature of such a national cost containment program. At the time President Nixon signed into law PL 93-222, the Health Maintenance Organization Act of 1973, it was hoped that by 1980 there would be a sufficient number of HMOs to enroll 90 percent of the U.S. population if they so desired. This hope clearly has not been met (Saward & Fleming, 1980). As of June 1980 approximately nine million persons belonged to 240 health maintenance organizations throughout the country (Saward & Fleming, 1980). These figures represent an increase of two and one-half million subscribers and 59 HMOs since a major HMO census five years ago (Wetherille & Nordley, 1975). Most indicators are that the number of health maintenance organizations will continue to expand rapidly and perhaps accelerate in the near future. For example, by the end of 1985 it is estimated that 15 percent of the greater Boston area population will belong to HMOs (Harvard Community Health Plan, 1980). At present about 25 percent of the people in Seattle, Washington belong to HMOs.

There are two major models for the organization of HMOs. One is called the medical foundation or individual practice association (IPA); the other, the prepaid group practice (PGP). Both types of HMOs are characterized by

103

the enrollment of a defined and voluntary population, the prepayment for care, and the provision of a wide variety of medical services only by those physicians who are hired by or contracted to the HMO. More simply stated, an HMO in general has a closed panel of physicians (providers) and a closed panel of patients (members).

In a number of other ways the IPA and prepaid group practice models differ considerably. An individual practice association often has as its providers fee-for-service physicians who, on the basis of a capitation arrangement, treat plan members in their own offices. This structure contrasts considerably with most prepaid group practice HMOs, which generally have a centralized health center and a salaried physician staff which often works only for the HMO. Although research by Roemer and Shonick (1973) indicates that group practice HMOs substantially reduce medical care expenditures, this reduction has not been demonstrated for the IPAs. There is some indication that by far the most substantial cost savings for group practice HMOs are found in the area of reduced hospital utilization (Gaus, Cooper, & Hirschman, 1976).

Mental Health Services

How are HMOs relevant to the provision of mental health services in this country? A central element in the 1973 HMO Act was a section describing the "basic health services" to be provided by HMOs seeking to be federally qualified. Federal qualification is of great value in a number of ways, the most important of which is that *any federally qualified HMO must be offered as an alternative to conventional health insurance by businesses in its service area with over 25 employees.* This "mandatory dual choice" provides qualified HMOs with greater access to potential members than was the case previously (Dorsey, 1975).

In order to be qualified, the HMO must provide "short-term (not to exceed 20 visits) outpatient evaluation and crisis intervention mental health services." The law is not specific as to which professions must provide these services, what constitutes a visit, and so on, and there has been considerable variation in the structure and format for delivery of HMO mental health treatment.

Levin and Glasser (1979) present survey data which strongly indicates that as of 1978 nearly all HMOs in one manner or another were seeking to provide mental health treatment. Sixty-eight percent of the operational HMOs they contacted responded to their questionnaires. Of these, 87 percent offered mental health coverage as part of their basic health plan. This is a major increase from a similar survey undertaken in 1976, which found that only 46 percent of the responding HMOs provided mental health services (Budman & Del Gaudio, 1979). It is clear that the total number of HMOs and the number that provide mental health treatment as part of their basic benefit package is increasing markedly.

Models of HMO Mental Health Services

Provision of mental health services to *all* members within an HMO is a relatively new phenomenon and might not have occurred to any significant degree were it not for the 1973 HMO legislation. Before then, the Southern California Permanente Medical Group, one of the largest HMOs in the country and the prototype for many others, offered mental health services as part of a "special" rider at an additional cost. With the increased legislative impetus for universal mental health coverage (for up to 20 outpatient visits), health maintenance organizations are exploring various models for the provision of high quality but affordable services.

Within prepaid group practice HMOs three models, or their variations, generally describe the manner in which mental health services are provided: a consultation model, an in-house direct service model, and an outside contractual direct service model. In the IPA-type HMO a psychotherapist would, like other physician providers, be paid on the basis of a capitation and/or co-payment arrangement.

Consultation Model

In the mental health consultation model, described by Coleman and Patrick (1978) at the Community Health Plan (CHP) in New Haven, Connecticut, mental health services are provided by the primary medical care staff. Although mental health professionals are available to provide direct services if necessary, most service is provided by physicians and nurses working in consultation with social workers. Ideally, there is no separation between who cares for the patient when he or she is physically ill and/or psychologically troubled. Furthermore, there is an orientation toward care of the total person, without the splitting off of particular types of care to specialists. In theory, at least, such a model for mental health services supports a primary practice orientation and moves away from the current trend of specialization in medical care. For a number of reasons this approach has not withstood the test of time, and mental health services at CHP are increasingly provided directly by mental health professionals (Schwartz, 1980).

A variety of factors mitigate against the broad establishment of this model. For one, not all physicians or nurses feel inclined to treat mental health problems, even with consultation. It is one thing to counsel a young male or female patient about the use of birth control, or to discuss diet with another patient. It is a completely different matter to deal with a seriously depressed or borderline psychotic patient. In addition, even those primary medical staff with a natural ability and inclination to be helpful may be seriously pressed for time. HMOs are typically very busy medical practices with large panels of patients being assigned to each provider. The opportunity for medical staff to provide even short-term counseling on a consistent basis is limited.

Brodsky (1970) supervised general practitioners and medical specialists enrolled in a course for doctors interested in conducting psychotherapy. Although this group of physicians was highly motivated, they tended to discontinue doing psychotherapy shortly after the course. Brodsky reported that they became uncomfortable with the complexities of therapy and anxious about dealing with patients whose symptoms increased or with whom it was difficult to communicate.

Another problem with the consultation model is that it can lead to a devaluation of the mental health therapist's role, accompanied by anger and resentment toward the mental health staff. If the medical staff believes that "therapy is a snap—all you need is a few easy leasons," then they may also begin to wonder why the health plan must support a number of expensive specialists in that area. In a setting where all staff is working long and hard but mental health staff drop by only occasionally to do consultation, then the latter come to be resented as "Monday morning quarterbacks."

In-House Direct Service Model

This model is described by Budman, Feldman, and Bennett (1979) as a program where an in-house staff of specialists comprised of psychiatrists, psychologists, social workers, and psychiatric nurses provides most of the direct care to patients with mental health problems who are referred by other medical specialists or by primary care staff.

Under a direct service model, mental health is generally viewed as one of a number of specialty care areas, such a surgery, obstetrics, and dentistry. Although there is an explicit differentiation of function between these specialty areas and primary care (i.e., internal medicine, family medicine, or pediatrics), there are also some significant unifying factors. For example, all medical care specialists and primary care staff treat patients directly. Thus, if health plan membership rises dramatically, everyone is equally affected by the influx. This contrasts sharply with the consultation model, where the consultative role to a great degree can be seen as insulating the mental health provider from the real-life exigencies of the health plan. In the direct service model all providers, specialists or not, are front-line troops. Furthermore, it is not infrequent for a specialist to become the primary focus of a patient's care. For example, a chronically disturbed patient in intermittent treatment with a mental health provider probably will have more planned and ongoing contact with that staff member than any other health care professional in the system. Under such circumstances the primary care/specialty care distinction breaks down.

Another unifying factor in such a model is that organization-wide structures for nurses and doctoral-level staff cut across specialty areas. Thus, psychologists and psychiatrists may join with M.D.s from other departments in a physician group. Psychiatric nurses presumably will be part of a plan-wide nursing group. At the Harvard Community Health Plan (HCHP) in Boston, each of the three separate full-service medical centers has a psychiatrist as its physician-in-chief. In addition, the director of nursing for the entire HCHP is a psychiatric nurse. Such a state of affairs would be most unlikely under a model which did not integrate the mental health staff with other medical staff.

Although this model gives up the continuity implied by a primary care team (physician/nurse) which provides all types of care (the goal in the consultative model), treatment is offered within one closed system and often in the same physical plant. Such physical proximity and organizational integration makes for easy referral and close working relationships between mental health and other staff.

Muller (1978) has several major criticisms of this model; lower staff "motivation" for the provision of good care, inferior "quality of care," a less distinctive identity for the mental health staff, and greater cost to the HMO than under the contractual service model. He gives no data or examples to support his position, and most of his points are cogently disputed by Bennett (1978). For example, in rebutting Muller's cost argument, Bennett states: "If cost to the HMO is less . . . , what about cost to the member? Capitation payments go further if fewer 'heads' show up" (p. 1249).

The direct service model is probably the most frequently applied in HMO mental health delivery at present. However, with the mushrooming of the health maintenance organization movement, other approaches such as the contractual model described below will certainly become increasingly common.

Outside Contractual Direct Service Model

This model entails the provision of mental health services to the HMO by a private, closed-panel group of mental health providers or autonomous individual providers contracted to the HMO to provide mental health care on the basis of a capitation or a fee-for-service arrangement. This model is favored by Muller (1978).

Under such an arrangement, an individual provider or groups of providers, or an entire community mental health center, may contract with the HMO to be the mental health service for HMO members. Services may be provided on a per capita prepaid arrangement, such as $12 per member (annual rate) paid to the contractor regardless of whether or not services are used, or on a fee-for-service basis using rates negotiated by the providers and the HMO. In some cases the arrangement combines aspects of prepaid and fee-for-service care, such as a patient co-payment arrangement.

One variation of this model can be a mental health IPA which contracts with the HMO for mental health services. This situation is well exemplified by the California Psychological Health Plan and the newly developing Massachusetts Psychological Health Plan, both of which are actually single-purpose IPAs which contract with other health plans or insurance companies to provide the mental health treatment.

These types of contractual arrangements have several benefits. Minimal start-up money is required for the HMO to begin offering mental health services. No mental health staff need be hired, no space needs to be rented, no support staff need be added. Additionally, the mental health practitioners involved in such an arrangement simply continue the work they are already doing and "add" HMO patients to their established practice.

There are major questions about whether this model will work as well as the in-house model. Under the contract model the mental health staff is only peripherally involved with the medical staff. They are very much separated from the goals, internal workings, and directions of the organization. If the contract with the providers is a capitation arrangement, fewer referrals mean less work. The contractor may intentionally or unintentionally build barriers to treatment and thereby meet the contractual requirements at the lowest cost and least effort. A fee-for-service or co-payment arrangement may not cost the HMO much directly, but it may cost the patient a great deal in additional out-of-pocket fees.

Further, this model allows little quality control. Under the in-house model, staff are carefully screened before hiring and their activities are closely supervised by others, usually more senior staff. In one variation of the contractual model any private practitioner of a particular discipline, such as a psychiatrist, may become a provider after an initial financial investment into the HMO. This allows for no uniformity of treatment patterns and little cost or quality control.

Although for the sake of clarity these three models for mental health service delivery in the HMO have been described as distinctive approaches, in the real world they tend not to exist in their "pure" forms. Frequently there is some variation which may combine aspects of two or more models. The most likely of these variations is probably an in-house direct service system which also emphasizes consultation to medical staff regarding mental health and patient management problems.

Unique Aspects of the HMO as a Mental Health Delivery System

A number of characteristics of the HMO make it a unique setting for the provision of mental health care. In this discussion of these characteristics, the reader should keep in mind that they apply mostly to the prepaid group practice (PGP) HMO. The medical foundation or independent practice association (IPA) may function considerably differently from the PGP and is distinct from the private practice of medicine only in its capitation arrangement.

Insofar as the HMO is a closed system—that is, a relatively fixed panel of providers supplying health care to a relatively fixed panel of patients for a relatively fixed pool of money—one is constantly faced with the challenges and opportunities inherent in making optimal use of finite resources. Although on a larger, national scale legislators and administrators may be faced with such choices, they are commonly less articulated because they involve competition among many organizationally different interest groups. Within a PGP HMO these resource decisions are part of everyday life for professional staff, administrators, and planners.

As Budman, Feldman, and Bennett (1979) discuss, the HMO health care system exists in a constant state of "dynamic tension." The three points of potentially divergent influence in this tension are the patient (member), the health care provider, and the system or health plan as a whole. Decisions regarding the type of health care provided and the overall benefit structure of a given HMO must take into account all three perspectives as well as the fact that resources within the system are finite.

The "dynamic tension" of the system and the finite pool of resources have important ramifications for the provision of mental health service within an HMO.

Limits to Choice and Breadth of Service

Unless a medical provider in an HMO is willing to suggest that a patient seek mental health services outside the HMO on a fee-for-service basis, the physician or nurse medical care provider *must* use the existing HMO mental health system for his or her patients. Obviously, this is in sharp contrast to the independent fee-for-service physician who can seek services for his or her patients from among available independent mental health providers or alternative agencies, such as a local community mental health center. The choice is only limited by the number and quality of mental health providers available. But the cost in this case is borne by the patient.

The limited choice available to HMO members means that the health plan must have a variety of mental health staff providing services (psychologists, psychiatrists, social workers, and psychiatric nurses). Furthermore, the ideal staff member should be flexible and skilled in a wide range of approaches and familiar with treating a variety of patients. For example, it would work poorly for an HMO mental health service to be staffed by one or two male psychiatrists familiar only with long-term individual psychoanalytic psychotherapy.

The limited choice of mental health providers available within the HMO would have very different implications were the HMO the only health service delivery system available to a particular population. Because HMOs are characterized by voluntary enrollment, the HMO system is always in competition with another form of service delivery or with another HMO. Thus, if a given HMO delivers poor quality health or mental health services, members may choose to leave the system and seek care elsewhere.

Close Accountability

The HMO closed panel system is much like a balloon: If one pinches it at one end, the other end expands. If mental health services are not being offered in a timely and reasonably high quality fashion by specialized mental health providers, there begins to back up into medical services a large number of patients who either are waiting to see a mental health provider or are disappointed with the specialized mental health care they received. Similarly, when medical services within the HMO are functioning poorly, the squeeze is felt in the mental health department via inappropriate referrals.

In a manner quite different from almost any other health care delivery system, an HMO forces a close linkage between health and mental health care. All aspects of the system are interdependent. Both mental health and medical care staff share the same organizational goals. Successes or failures in the provision of quality care are shared by all.

A Brief Therapy Model and Continuity of Care

As well as being a source of health care services, an HMO is also an insurance company. Throughout the HMO there is an emphasis upon timely and cost-effective care. As fully discussed elsewhere (Budman, 1981) a myth has developed in this country that psychotherapy must be long-term and continuous in order to be effective. Research findings regarding the efficacy of psychotherapy have failed to demonstrate that brief treatment is any less effective than long-term therapy.

There is an emphasis upon brief therapy in the HMO because new patients are continually entering the mental health subsystem. All such patients must be treated in a timely and cost-effective manner or the mental health subsystem will become a bottleneck and the flow of patients will grind to a halt. The HMO must provide prepaid mental health care without extended waiting lists and without the use of referral to non-HMO providers. These challenges have led most HMOs to provide brief therapy to most members, while a small percentage of patients requiring long-term care are treated on a continuing basis (Bennett & Wisneski, 1979).

Indeed, the HMO is an ideal setting for the provision of what has been called "discontinuous psychotherapy"; that is, several courses of brief therapy over an extended period of time (Budman, 1981). Cummings and VandenBos (1979) provide an excellent example of such discontinuous therapy.

The HMO is well suited for the provision of brief discontinuous psychotherapy because patients do have a continuing relationship with the primary care providers of the HMO and with the HMO as an organization. Thus, a patient may complete a course of short-term group therapy with a particular mental health provider, but the patient remains a member of the HMO system as a whole, thus facilitating an "institutional transference." This transference may be most helpful in maintaining continuity of care even if a specialized mental health provider is seen only rarely (Budman & Clifford, 1979).

Preventive Mental Health Services

Because prevention is cost-effective, such programs may have exceptional benefits within the HMO framework. A basic premise of the HMO is that maintaining health is cheaper than treating more serious illness. Therefore, some HMOs have devoted time and money to programs described as "health education" or lifestyle change programs. These are not necessarily run by mental health specialists, but it is not uncommon for psychological issues to be prominent in such programs. For example, Tongas (1979), a psychologist at the Permanente Medical Group in Southern California, developed a large-scale smoking cessation program. At the Harvard Community Health Plan in Boston for the past five years we have been examining the utility of a preventive psychoeducational group approach for HMO members undergoing the stresses of marital separation (Wertlieb & Budman, 1981). Sank and his colleagues (1979) at the George Washington University Health Plan preventively treated groups of plan members who had been taken hostage by the Hanafi Moslems when they took over the B'nai Brith building in Washington, D.C. in 1977.

Opportunities for Research

Since the late 1960s interest has grown in studying the impact which the provision of mental health services has upon the utilization of other health care services. In their landmark study at the Permanente Medical Group, Follette and Cummings (1967) found that brief psychotherapeutic intervention appears to have a major "offset" effect. That is, for distressed patients seen by mental health therapists, even for one or two sessions, there was a substantial and long-lasting reduction in their subsequent use of other health care services (Cummings & Follette, 1976). At present, this area of research, called "offset" or "impact" studies, has gained major importance and has been the topic of two reviews (Schlesinger, Mumford, & Glass, 1980; Jones & Vischi, 1979) and one international conference (ADAMHA Conference on the impact of alcohol, drug and mental health intervention upon the use of medical care services, October 15-17, 1980). Of the approximately 15 offset studies conducted to date, the vast majority have taken place in HMO settings. This research opportunity is due to the fact that the HMO database provides an excellent location for examining pre- to post-mental health intervention changes in health care utilization. Chapter 14 in this volume discusses in greater depth the findings of such research and their methodological problems.

The HMO is also ideally suited to be a study site for health care utilization changes after life stress (Wertlieb & Budman, 1981). Finally, because the patient population base is relatively stable, longitudinal psychotherapy outcome research studies can also be implemented at such health plans (Budman, Demby, & Randall, 1980).

Conclusions

There has been enormous growth in HMOs throughout this country during the past decade. The promise of the 1980s is one of continued and expanded growth of such health plans. This chapter has described the structure of health maintenance organizations, alternative models for mental health services within such settings, and some of the unique opportunities for linkage which such settings provide. In many ways, HMOs represent a microcosm and a living laboratory in which the interface between health and mental health services may be examined. Undoubtedly, in the years ahead new programs will be tried in which more and more mental health professionals and behavioral scientists will be asked to play significant roles.

References

Bennett, M. J. Mental health services in HMOs. *American Journal of Psychiatry,* 1978, 135, 1249.

Bennett, M. J., & Wisneski, M. J. Continuous psychotherapy within an HMO. *American Journal of Psychiatry,* 1979, 136, 1283-1287.

Brodsky, C. M. The systemic incompatibility of medical practice and psychotherapy. *Diseases of the Nervous System,* 1970, 31, 597-604.

Budman, S. H. (Ed.). *Forms of brief therapy.* New York: Guilford Press, 1981.

Budman, S. H., & Clifford, M. Short-term group therapy for couples in a health maintenance organization. *Professional Psychology,* 1979, 10, 419-429.

Budman, S. H., & Del Gaudio, A. C. A survey of psychologists at health maintenance organizations and community mental health centers. *Professional Psychology,* 1979, 10, 244-248.

Budman, S. H., Bennett, M. J., & Wisneski, M. J. Short-term group psychotherapy: An adult developmental model. *International Journal of Group Psychotherapy,* 1980, 30, 63-76.

Budman, S. H., Bennett, M. J., & Wisneski, M. J. An adult developmental model of short-term group psychotherapy. In S. H. Budman (Ed.), *Forms of brief therapy.* New York: Guilford Press, 1981.

Budman, S. H., Demby, A., & Randall, M. Short-term group therapy: Who succeeds? Who fails? *Group,* 1980, 4, 3-16.

Budman, S. H., Feldman, J., & Bennett, M. J. Adult mental health services in a health maintenance organization. *American Journal of Psychiatry,* 1979, 136, 392-395.

Coleman, J. V., & Patrick, D. D. Psychiatry and general health care. *American Journal of Public Health,* 1978, 68, 451-457.

Cummings, N. A. Prolonged (ideal) versus short-term (realistic) psychotherapy. *Professional Psychology,* 1977, 8, 491-501.

Cummings, N. A., & Follette, W. T. Brief psychotherapy and medical utilization. In H. Dorken (Ed.), *The professional psychologist today.* San Francisco: Jossey-Bass, 1976.

Cummings, N. A., & VandenBos, G. R. The general practice of psychology. *Professional Psychology,* 1979, 10, 430-440.

Dorsey, J. L. The Health Maintenance Organization Act of 1973 (PL 93-222) and prepaid group practice plans. *Medical Care,* 1975, 13, 1-9.

Follette, W. T., & Cummings, N. A. Psychiatric services and medical utilization in a prepaid health plan setting. *Medical Care,* 1967, 5, 25-35.

Gaus, C. R., Cooper, B. S., & Hirschman, C. G. Contrasts in HMO and fee-for-service performance. *Social Security Bulletin,* May 1976, 3-14. DHEW Publication No. (SSA) 76-11700.

Harvard Community Health Plan. HMO's in Boston (internal document), 1980.

Jones, K. R., & Vischi, T. Impact of alcohol, drug abuse, and mental health treatment on medical care utilization. *Medical Care,* 1979, 17 (Supplement).

Levin, B. L., & Glasser, J. H. A survey of mental health service coverage within health maintenance organizations. *American Journal of Public Health,* 1979, 69, 1120-1125.

Muller, D. J. The external provision of health maintenance organization mental health services. *American Journal of Psychiatry,* 1978, 135, 735-738.

Roemer, M. I., & Shonick, W. HMO performance: The recent evidence. *Milbank Memorial Fund Quarterly,* 1973, 51, 271-317.

Saward, E. W., & Fleming, S. Health maintenance organizations. *Scientific American,* 1980, 243, 47-54.

Sank, L. I. Primary prevention and treatment in a health maintenance organization. *American Psychologist,* 1979, 34, 334-338.

Schlesinger, H., Mumford, E., & Glass, G. V. The effects of psychological intervention on recovery from surgery. In F. Guerra & J. A. Aldrete (Eds.), *Emotional and psychological responses to anesthesia and surgery.* New York: Grune and Stratton, 1980.

Schwartz, M. Personal communication, September 11, 1980.

Tongas, P. N. The Kaiser Permanente Smoking Control Program: Its purpose and implications for an HMO. *Professional Psychology,* 1979, 10, 409-418.

Wetherille, R. L., & Nordley, J. M. A census of HMO's, April 1975. Minneapolis, MN: Interstudy, 1975.

Wertlieb, D., & Budman, S. H. The health-mental health linkage: Mandates and challenges for program evaluation research. In W. Tosh & J. Stahler (Eds.), *Innovative approaches to mental health evaluation.* New York: Academic Press, 1981.

7

Mental Health Providers in Primary Care Settings

Donald Wertlieb

*Eliot-Pearson Department of Child Study,
Tufts University*

As health care providers, planners, and policy makers confront the challenge of the "primary care priority" in national health care delivery, increasing attention is being paid to health-mental health "linkages," "interfaces," or "interdigitations." Considerable excitement and controversy surrounds the efforts of traditional mental health disciplines to define their roles, broaden their influence, justify their input, and demonstrate their effectiveness and necessity in the emerging health care system. These efforts involve significant conceptual and scientific revitalizations and reorientations, many of which can be subsumed under the umbrella discipline of "behavioral medicine" (Matarazzo, 1980; Schwartz & Weiss, 1977). Further, these efforts are dependent upon advances toward a deeper understanding of health and illness and upon advances in associated technologies only recently subjected to scientific scrutiny. As is often the case, public policy on primary care must be formulated before all the relevant scientific data can be accrued. At the same time, important developments are underway. This chapter reviews those developments and efforts involving the role of mental health providers (MHP) in primary care settings. Of particular concern are the contributions of consultation-liaison psychiatrists and health care psychologists. In addition to this overview, a framework for identifying MHP contributions and roles in primary care settings is presented. Diagnostic, therapeutic, teaching, and research functions are delineated as they affect patients, primary care providers (PCP), and the health care system. Comments on some of the problems and obstacles in fulfilling these roles are also considered.

The Primary Care Priority

Since the early 1970s, a top priority of federal health planners has been to strengthen primary health care delivery systems—that is, the "first contact" level of health services. Typically, primary care refers to ambulatory care by general internists, family practitioners, and pediatricians, although other specialties may function as primary care providers, including obstetrics-gynecology and even psychiatry (Oken & Fink, 1976). An Institute of Medicine (1978) report characterized primary care as "accessible, comprehensive, coordinated and continual care provided by accountable providers of health services." This and a subsequent report (Institute of Medicine, 1979) elaborated upon these five essential attributes as follows:

(1) *Accessibility of care* refers to the provider's responsibility to assist patients or potential patients to overcome temporal, spatial, economic, and psychologic barriers to health care. . . .

(2) *Comprehensiveness of care* refers to the willingness and ability of providers to handle the great majority of health problems arising in the populations served. . . . His or her services are not restricted by concentration on [a particular] specialty.

(3) *Coordination of care* denotes the primary care practitioner's role as ombudsman, coordinating the total care—including that provided by specialists—of his or her patients. . . .

(4) *Continuity of care* depends largely on the first three attributes of primary care, requiring *active* commitment on the practitioner's part to maintaining an ongoing relationship with each patient.

(5) *Accountability* requires that primary care providers review regularly both the process and outcomes of care with attention to potential improvement, and also entails commitment to ensuring that patients are informed decision-makers [p. 6].

In discussing primary care, Alpert and Charney (1974) wrote:

[The] primary care doctor spends most of his time thinking about the patient and the impact of various forces on his health or illness over a period of time. The secondary or tertiary level doctor spends most of his time thinking about a disease state or a technical skill and how various patients fit into or alter that field of interest over a period of time. For one, the illness is the episode; for the other, the patient is the episode [p. 3].

These requirements for holism, comprehensiveness, and continuity mandate significant reorientations in the health care delivery associated with a number of converging factors, some of which are listed below.

(1) A disaffection with current medical care both in terms of quality and cost (Illich, 1976; Mechanic, 1979; Rogers, 1977; Wildavsky, 1977).

(2) Greater awareness of "new morbidity" (Haggerty, Roghmann, & Pless, 1975), or health problems where behavioral, lifestyle, and psychosocial factors are as important as or more important than traditional medical concerns with infectious disease (Eisenberg, 1977a, 1977b; Rachman & Philips, 1980; Stachnik, 1980).

(3) Rediscovery of the health-mental health linkage—that is, the preponderance of emotional problems in patients presenting in general medical practice and high medical utilization patterns by psychiatric patients (e.g., Hankin & Oktay, 1979; Mumford, Schlesinger, & Glass, 1979; Regier, Goldberg, & Taube, 1978; Wertlieb & Budman, 1981).

(4) Greater appreciation of health and illness as biopsychosocial phenomena, along with an emphasis on holistic approaches, prevention and health maintenance, and connections between life stress and illness (e.g., Cobb, 1976; Cohen, 1979; Engle, 1977, 1980; Lipowski, 1977a, 1977b; Pelletier, 1979; Smilkstein, 1980; Wertlieb, 1979).

(5) Advances in conceptualizing, understanding, and studying those factors listed in 2, 3, and 4 above, including Engel's (1977, 1980) biopsychosocial model, the new psychosomatics (Lipowski, 1977a, 1977b), and the preventive health paradigm (Wertlieb, 1979).

Addressing these problems and applying these understandings involves new challenges for mental health care providers and primary care providers. The mental health disciplines (psychiatry, psychology, social work, and psychiatric nursing) must become more aware of their importance and influence in the general health care system. PCPs must become more cognizant of significant mental health issues affecting their practice. These areas of common concern include addressing emotional or psychiatric problems presented by patients, gathering a sufficiently comprehensive history for accurate diagnosis, developing treatment plans and interventions encompassing the relevant biopsychosocial factors of the patient's problem, and maintaining the patient's compliance with therapeutic regimens or health maintenance protocols. By nature of his or her training, the MHP also brings additional education relevant to the primary care setting, such as skills and experience in psychological or psychosomatic diagnosis and therapy. The MHP's skills in interpersonal relations can enhance the functioning of the primary care setting, either in terms of the PCP-patient relationship or collegial relationships among the multidisciplinary PCP team. Many MHPs trained in the scientist-practitioner model—usually clinical psychologists or psychiatrists—can also bring their research skills to bear upon the problems of the primary care setting through basic or applied research, including program evaluation.

Meeting the primary care priority requires interdisciplinary collaboration, particularly active participation by MHPs. The nature and scope of this participation are articulated below, emphasizing roles of consultation-liaison psychiatry and health care psychology. Similar descriptions could be generated for other traditional MHP disciplines, such as psychiatric nursing and social work (e.g., Nason & Delbanco, 1976; Rittelmeyer & Flynn, 1978). However, some of the particular issues relevant to such an articulation are beyond the scope of the present chapter. Nevertheless, the framework presented below does have general application for all MHPs in primary care settings.

Consultation-Liaison Psychiatry

According to one of its major proponents,

> consultation-liaison psychiatry represents application of the psychosomatic approach to clinical work. Its hallmark is the gathering and applying of information from several levels of abstraction relevant to patient care. Its basic assumption is that an integrated approach results in optimal health care, one sensitive to peoples' needs, mindful of prevention, and economically sound [Lipowski, 1974: 626].

Lipowski recognizes that

> psychiatrists can only modestly contribute to such care. Their major function is to demonstrate that it can be done and how. . . . .Psychiatrists should aim deliberately at assuming the role of integrating health care and mediating between overspecialized physicians on the one hand and the psychosocially oriented but medically naive behavioral scientists on the other [p. 626].

The development of consultation-liaison psychiatry over the past fifty years has been traced by Lipowski (1967a, 1967b, 1974, 1975, 1977a,

1977b), Abram (1977), Enelow (1981), and Krakowski (1977). The history of articulating psychiatry's role in primary care settings is a shorter one, a newer effort responsive to the national health care priorities discussed above. This "specialization" of consultation-liaison psychiatry has been well chronicled and described by Abram (1977), Barksy (1980), Goldberg, Haas, Eaton, and Grubbs (1976), and Fink (1981). Although these discussions will not be repeated here, they do contribute to the framework for MHP participation in primary care settings presented in this chapter.

Health Care Psychology

"Health [care] psychology is the aggregate of the specific educational, scientific and professional contributions of the discipline of psychology to the promotion and maintenance of health, the prevention and treatment of illness, the identification of etiologic and diagnostic correlates of health, illness, and related dysfunction" (Matarazzo, 1980: 815). This definition is partly a response to the primary care priority and the related factors outlined above. It subsumes the more familiar specialization of clinical psychology, placing this mental health discipline in a more appropriate context of health as a biopsychosocial phenomenon. The subspecializations of medical psychology and pediatric psychology are similarly subsumed.

In some ways newer than its counterpart in medicine and psychiatry (i.e., consultation-liaison psychiatry), health care psychology claims it began almost seventy years ago. John B. Watson, to many the father of American psychology, wrote in 1912:

> The medical student must be taught that no matter whether he is specializing in surgery, obstetrics, or psychiatry, his subjects are human beings and not merely objects on which he may demonstrate his skill. This shift in his ideas of value will lead him to feel the need of psychologic training and to accept that training [p. 917].

A few years later, on the same issue of medical education, Bott (1928) argued that it was necessary for the medical student

> to think not in terms of special organs or organ systems but of the whole living organism as a person, reacting physically and mentally to a changing environment primarily social in character. . . . The conception of a living personality has to be given to students and kept alive in their minds at the same time as they are studying the physical structure and processes of the human body [p. 292].

The affinity with the earlier citied manifesto on primary care by Alpert and Charney (1974) is both remarkable and heartening.

These early declarations by Watson and Bott serve as a starting point for Stone et al.'s (1979) account of the historical development of health care psychology. These early concerns foreshadow some of the major domains of modern health care psychology. The impetus for such development derives from the collaboration between pediatricians and psychologists, a "new marriage" described by Kagan (1965), bearing the new discipline "pediatric psychology" (Wright, 1967, 1979). Statements by Schofield (1969, 1979) and the American Psychological Association Task Force on Health Research (1976) are also seminal in the emergence of health care psychology and provide the historical tracings necessary in defining the discipline.

MHP Roles and Functions
in Primary Care Settings

Traditionally, psychiatrists' and psychologists' service functions have involved mostly direct and indirect provision of mental health services. This is certainly the case in such specialty settings as psychiatric hospitals, psychiatric units in general hospitals, community mental health centers, and the fee-for-service mental health clinics. These settings rely heavily on interdisciplinary teamwork, with the traditional mental health professions collaborating in patient care. Teaching activities generally involve exchange of expertise among these mental health professionals. Research in these settings is most often focused on basic and applied mental health issues.

With the integration of the MHP into primary health care, there is broadening, elaboration, and differentiation of roles and functions. The basic involvement remains in diagnosis, treatment, teaching, and research. However, the focus moves beyond that of emotional disturbance and mental illness, broadening to include health and illness in the biopsychosocial framework referenced above. Indeed, the patient's own statement of the problem is most likely to be of a nonpsychiatric nature and presented to a PCP rather than an MHP. Interdisciplinary teamwork is central to work in primary care settings, but rather than the mental health team (psychiatrist, psychologist, social worker, psychiatric nurse), the MHP collaborates with pediatricians, family practitioners, internists, nurse practitioners, medical nurses, and medical social workers. Teaching activities involve the presentation of mental health concepts and skills to non-mental health professionals. Research takes a biopsychosocial perspective, rather than the narrow mental health or psychiatric focus in mental health settings. In primary care settings, the MHP continues his or her usual mental health services but broadens his or her activities in accordance with the comprehensive, integrated biopsychosocial orientation of primary care.

The nature, variety, and significance of mental health contributions to primary care settings can be articulated within the framework suggested in Table 7.1. Diagnostic, therapeutic, teaching, and research functions of the MHP can be described in terms of the target or focus of the MHP's efforts. Some of these activities are "case-centered"—that is, focused upon the patient and/or the patient's family. Other activities are directed toward the individual PCP or primary care team and are thus "consultee-centered." Meyer and Mendelson's (61) concept of the "operational group" emphasizes the consultant's role in the medical team as "enabler of interpersonal communication, interpreter of the patient's behavior, and reducers of disruptive conflict" (Lipowski, 1967a: 166). Still other functions are "systems-centered," focusing on change in the health care system, often on a global level. Of course, these differentiations of target and focus are overlapping and useful mainly as conceptual tools. Indeed, there are few, if any, MHP activities which could be said to reflect only one of these categories.

It may be that the capacity to maintain these multiple perspectives on any single activity or function serves to enhance effectiveness of the MHP in primary care settings. That is, awareness of these various levels and their complex interactions should be part of an MHP's conceptualization of his or her role. An MHP may emphasize one or another subset of the functions or targets presented in Table 7.1. For instance, only service functions, such as diagnosis and treatment, may be performed by a particular pediatric psychologist, or a psychiatrist may provide only consultee-centered teaching in a seminar in a primary care setting, or a social psychologist may restrict his or her activities to research on patient compliance with physician recommendations. In any event, the scheme presented in Table 7.1 serves to outline current potential contributions of MHPs in primary care settings, as further described below.

Diagnosis

The MHP contributes to the generation and integration of data leading to a biopsychosocial diagnosis of a patient's illness, disease, or "dis-ease." At some stage in the diagnostic process the MHP serves as the proponent of the psychological or psychosocial perspective, at risk for "overpsychologizing" the situation or reifying a mind-body dichotomy which ultimately needs to be overcome. As Brill (1975) notes, "the task is to reconcile the medical-

TABLE 7.1   Mental Health Provider Contributions to Primary Care

	FOCUS		
Function	*Case-Centered: Patient and Family as Target*	*Consultee-Centered: PCP and Operational Group as Target*	*System-Centered: Health Care System as Target*
Diagnosis	contribute to data base and integration of biopsychosocial diagnosis of illness	encourage and model holistic, biopsychosocial approach to patient assessment interpret patient patient behavior to PCP	implement health assessment and screening to identify patients at biopsychosocial risks
Treatment	provide guidance and/or brief psychotherapy develop and implement management and treatment plans addressing behavioral and psychosocial dimensions of patient care	encourage and model holistic, biopsychosocial approach to patient care enable communication and teamwork among PCP team liaison to psychiatric or other specialty services	implement psychoeducational, lifestyle, or health education services; e.g., smoking or weight control
Teaching	reframe and relate symptoms to lifestyle factors, behavior, stress, etc. at rounds, case conferences, teaching conferences	didactic interaction regarding doctor-patient relationship, interviewing, diagnosis and treatment of emotional disorders, human development	implement integrated behavioral sciences curriculum in medical school, teaching hospital, or continuing education
Research	refine diagnostic criteria in a biopsychosocial framework basic research in etiology of illness and health	identify PCP behaviors associated with patient compliance with treatment regimen develop diagnostic and treatment protocols which address biopsychosocial aspects of illness	program evaluation cost-offset research quality assurance

biological approach with the psychosocial one and to somehow present this comprehensive view in a practical and meaningful way in the medical setting" (p. 113).

Lipowski (1976b) offers five categories of differential diagnostic problems faced by the MHP and primary care team:

(1) psychological presentation of organic disease,

(2) psychological complications of organic disease,

(3) psychological reactions to organic disease,

(4) somatic presentation of psychiatric disorders,

(5) "psychosomatic" disorders.

This classification is useful only to the extent that it does not lead the provider or the patient to an overly facile, overly simplified, non-integrated appreciation of the patient's problem. Indeed, "if one views disease from a multicausal point of view, every disorder can be considered psychosomatic, since every disorder is affected in some fashion by emotional factors" (Kaplan, 1980: 1973).

Feldman (1978) and Martin (1980) point to the development of the psychosocial history as a crucial component of the diagnostic process in primary care, a component often dependent upon direct or indirect care efforts by the MHP.

> Despite an emphasis on the teaching of the relationship between illness and the patient's emotional status internists have a tendency to minimize psychiatric issues. Even when significant emotional difficulties are present, physicians tend to place these near the end of their problem-oriented lists. It is common for the internist to note the pain and stiffness of degenerative arthritis, chronic obesity, and other overt symptoms before noting depression or anxiety [Martin, 1980: 2031].

Whether through direct intervention with the patient and family or through indirect consultation with the PCP, the MHP can encourage and model a holistic biopsychosocial approach to patient assessment. Part of this process often involves interpretation of patient behavior to the PCP, increasing the PCP's awareness of meanings beyond the overt verbal content of the presentation. The PCP can be directed toward greater appreciation of sources of anxiety and depression for the patient and how they may or may not influence his or her illness behavior or complaints. This appreciation involves considerably more than identification of so-called psychosomatic or stress symptoms (such as tension headaches or low back pain). Rather, a biopsychosocial framework for understanding the symptoms, the patient's experience of the symptoms, and the patient's expectations, wishes, and fears within the PCP-patient relationship must be developed via the diagnostic process. For example, recognizing the need for new and revised diagnostic and screening instruments in medical settings, Millon, Green and Meagher (1979) have presented the Millon Behavioral Health Inventory (MBHI). This 150-item, self-report inventory shows some promise in facilitating the biopsychosocial diagnostic process in primary care.

As the kind of MHP-PCP diagnostic teamwork suggested above entrenches itself in a setting or system, alterations in the system itself are likely. For instance, prior to such collaboration, descriptions of the patient population served may underestimate the prevalence or significance of depression, anxiety, or other psychosocial or behavioral problems. With such collaborations, these problems may be more accurately recognized and diagnosed, or even overestimated. Depending on the degree of integration and type of care delivery system, one possible change could be an increased referral to psychiatric or social service components of the system. The MHP must maintain such a system-centered focus in order to have a perspective on the mental health contribution to the diagnostic activity of the setting.

Another system-centered contribution by MHPs in primary care settings is the implementation of health assessment and screening programs aimed at the identification of patients "at risk" (Wertlieb & Budman, 1981). The Kaiser-Permanente Multiphasic Health Appraisal is one such program being developed in a health maintenance organization (Harrington, 1978). By screening for particular behaviors, lifestyle patterns, or other health status indicators, the PCP can direct patients toward appropriate preventively oriented intervention programs. Further, identification of at-risk subpopulations within a patient population can focus and foster development of specialized interventions addressing their particular needs. Cigarette smoking, problem drinking, and overeating, for example, are behaviors which should alert the PCP and the system to potential health problems and a need for timely intervention.

Treatment

The value of screening and identifying patients "at risk" is related to the range of activities available for the treatment of these patients. That PCPs are indeed attempting to treat those patients who exhibit emotional disturbance is evidenced by the high, and often inappropriate, rate of prescribing of tranquilizing drugs (Eisenberg, 1977b). A literature survey by Hankin (1979) indicates that between 29 and 79 percent of primary care patients whose emotional disturbance may or may not be diagnosed receive a prescription for psychoactive drugs. About 70 percent of psychotropic drugs are prescribed by nonpsychiatrists (Kline, 1974). Again, the treatment contributions of the MHP in primary care settings can be considered from case-centered, consultee-centered, and system-centered perspectives, as suggested in Table 7.1.

As in the diagnostic process, the treatment process is potentially enhanced by the broadened biopsychosocial perspective fostered by the MHP. The MHP, in collaboration with the PCP team, develops and implements treatment and management plans addressing behavioral and psychosocial dimensions of patient care as well as biomedical dimensions. Kaplan (1980) calls such interventions "psychomedical treatment"—that is, an approach that emphasizes the interrelation of mind and body in the genesis of symptom and disorder (p. 1973).

The MHP in primary care settings is often called upon to provide psychotherapeutic services not unlike those provided in specialty mental health settings. Two major distinctions between traditional psychotherapy and that done in primary care settings represent appropriate accommodations to the demands of such settings; a shift toward brief therapies (see Budman, 1981), and an increased use of psychoeducational or guidance interventions (see Wertlieb, 1979; Wright, 1979). Many of these latter interventions recognize the value and importance of providing information and support conducive to a patient's carrying out responsibility for his or her own care in an active rather than passive manner.

Another accommodation has been the emergence of episodic psychotherapeutic treatment (Cummings & VandenBos, 1979). Just as primary medical care involves relatively brief encounters between patient and PCP over a number of years, so does the psychotherapy relationship take shape in such settings. Jacobson (1979) has described this "extensive therapy" and noted the reorientation it requires for the MHP.

A successful outcome of specialty mental health service typically has been based on the expectation that the patient will not return after the completion of psychotherapeutic intervention. The definition of successful outcome in primary care is quite the opposite: the PCP assumes that patients will continue to return for health care as needed. Thus, the MHP might employ a "string of beads" approach, in which the patient would work on a theme in a succession

of crisis episodes for which he or she would return to the same therapist to pick
up the treatment. The treatment course in this approach is not terminated but is
considered to have dormant phases [Institute of Medicine, 1979: 126].

An advantage of such approaches is a wider availability of such psychotherapy to more people at lower costs. Disadvantages include the relative dearth
of training for MHPs at this point for such therapy, as well as the possible
exclusion of patient populations in need of more intensive and time-
concentrated services. Furthermore, the effectiveness of such brief task-
centered treatment remains an important empirical question (Budman,
1981). However, there are significant indications that psychotherapy has an
extremely important role to play in the health care system (e.g., Mumford et
al., 1979; Olbrisch, 1977; Schlesinger, Mumford, & Glass, 1981; Wertlieb
& Budman, 1981).

Besides providing direct psychotherapeutic services to patients, the MHP
can have important impact via services to the PCP. Again, encouragement
and modeling of holistic biopsychosocial approaches are central. Capitaliz-
ing upon his or her training in human relations and interpersonal communication, the MHP can enable and facilitate communication and teamwork
among the PCP team as well as that between the patient and team. This
function of the MHP is emphasized by Bibring (1956), Kahana, (1959), and
Krakowski (1977). For instance, the MHP helps the consultee, the PCP,
"utilize the strength of his [PCP] personality in cooperatively [with the
patient] combatting illness" (Kahana, 1959).

The contemporary physician has been characterized as an impersonal,
uncaring, but technically skilled scientist (Martin, 1980). This indictment
may be less the case in primary care specialties than in others. Nonetheless,
this issue is one of special import for the MHP in primary care treatment. If
there is any truth to the saying that "90% of curing is caring," then the MHP
is in an excellent position to shift the attentions of the PCP to that important
"90%."

A specific contribution of the MHP to the PCP team is the traditional
liaison function. The MHP often holds the key to successful referral for
psychiatric services or other appropriate services in secondary, tertiary, or
other specialty areas of the health care system. This aspect of comprehensive
treatment should not be underemphasized. There is considerable evidence
that this component of primary care services needs improvement. Carey and
Kogan (1971) describe the complex factors involved in decision-making and
success around mental health referrals by PCPs.

Again, the proliferation and success of these case-centered and
consultee-centered treatment activities can significantly alter the health care

system. Further, some MHP activity can begin to focus upon the system level. For instance, given the mental health assessment and screening activities mentioned above, MHPs will have to develop and implement a range of treatment interventions tailored to address the identified risk factors. Psychoeducational, lifestyle, and/or health education groups centered on such issues as smoking, weight control, and psychosocial stress are among such interventions. For example, relaxation training can help with the stresses of job pressures; peer support groups may help people cope with the stresses of marital disruption (Harrington, 1978; Wertlieb, 1979). The MHP can make significant contributions to these types and level of services in primary care settings. Furthermore, as will be discussed below, training PCPs in the provision of such services or appropriate referral considerations, and evaluating such programs, constitutes major teaching and research functions for the MHP in primary care settings.

Teaching

Freedman and Sack (1979) suggest that "education is perhaps the greatest contribution psychiatry can give to primary care physicians" (p. 4). Wexler (1976) suggests that the behavioral sciences, particularly psychology, should "develop a model of the doctor's job and clothe it with the basic and essential information required for primary patient care" (p. 275). Again, it is useful to consider direct and indirect teaching services with case-centered, consultee-centered, and system-centered foci.

Though teaching would generally be considered a mutual exchange between the PCP and MHP, there are contributions by the MHP that more directly center upon the primary care patient and the patient's family. These contributions are generally related to the direct treatment of the patient but should also be acknowledged as didactic or teaching interventions. For instance, the MHP on a primary care team may be responsible for helping the patient reframe or relate symptoms to lifestyle factors, behavior, or stress. This same educational effort can be extended by the MHP in patient rounds or case conferences centered upon a particular patient, thus providing case-centered teaching to the PCP.

In terms of the consultee-centered focus—that is, teaching functions within the operational group—the MHP can rely significantly on didactic presentations on topics ranging from the doctor-patient relationship to interviewing techniques to the diagnosis and treatment of emotional disorders. Such content material is presented in recently published handbooks and textbooks (Freedman, Sack & Berger, 1979; Rosen, Geyman, & Layton, 1980; West, 1979). Matching mental health curricula with the interests and needs of the PCP team is a complicated and challenging task only recently yielding fruitful advances (e.g., Authier, 1979; Bibace & Walsh, 1979).

Much of this teaching activity occurs in the operational group, or health care team. However, there is now widespread recognition of the need to develop and implement integrated mental health and behavioral sciences curricula throughout the training and service delivery system, including medical school, teaching hospitals, residency programs, and continuing education settings (Bibace & Walsh, 1979; Wexler, 1976; Zuckerman, Carper, & Alpert, 1978). Such system-centered work by the MHP may be the most relevant and significant contribution to meeting the primary care mandate.

Besides those teaching efforts that transmit a mental health perspective and knowledge to the other members of the PCP team, there is a critical mandate for MHPs working in primary care settings to train members of their own discipline, to enable the next generation of health care psychologists or consultation-liaison psychiatrists to function more effectively. Thus, within-discipline teaching at the predoctoral and postdoctoral levels is important.

Research

The research orientation, skill, and activity of many MHPs are often considered among their most important contributions to primary care. Shepherd (1979) suggests that clinical investigation is a "logical point of entry for the psychiatrist in search of a necessary if not sufficient role on the primary care scene" (p. 222). Recent reviews of consultation-liaison psychiatry include growing attention to the research function (Lipowski, 1974; Enelow, 1981). Barksy (1980) urges that mental health providers should give

> highest priority to generating rigorous clinical research. This will form an intellectual and academic foundation beneath the psychiatric aspects of primary care. . . . It is precisely because psychiatry comes closest of all the specialties to addressing the total patient that it has an opportunity to be pivotal in the future of primary care medicine, and in the translation of behavioral science findings into medical and psychiatric practice [p. 227].

The American Psychological Association Task Force on Health Research (1976) notes:

> There is probably no specialty field within psychology that cannot contribute to the discovery of behavioral variables crucial to a full understanding of

susceptibility to physical illness, adaptation to such illness, and prophylactically motivated behaviors. The areas open to psychological investigation range from health care practices and health care delivery systems to the management of acute and chronic illness and to the psychology of medication and pain [p. 272].

As suggested in Table 7.1, research contributions by MHPs to primary care can include case-centered, consultee-centered, and system-centered targets. There are numerous research questions relating to the refinement of diagnostic criteria within a biopsychosocial framework. Empirical questions and problems abound on the etiology and treatment of illness. The preventive health paradigm (Wertlieb, 1979) raises such research issues as the identification of vulnerable populations and risk factors, the application and evaluation of psychological interventions aimed at decreasing illness and subsequent medical services utilization, and the enhancement of health and positive coping skills.

At the consultee-centered level, research efforts by MHPs may focus on the identification of PCP behaviors associated with improved patient compliance with treatment regimens. Other research efforts could address the development of diagnostic and treatment protocols which integrate the biopsychosocial aspects of illness.

At the system-centered level, program evaluation research is a major avenue for MHP participation in primary care. In particular, research on the "cost-offset effect" shows promise for a better conceptual and economic foundation for health-mental health linkages (Wertlieb & Budman, 1981, also see Chapter 4 of this volume for a more complete review of the "cost-offset effect"). The development of quality assurance methodologies represents another example of applied research of particular relevance to primary care.

Problems and Prospects

In carrying out any subset of the functions described above, the MHP will confront numerous obstacles and resistances, representing both personal and systemic issues. Articulation of these myriad issues is especially well handled in discussions by Barsky (1980), Fink (1981), Jacobson (1979), Lipowski (1977a, 1977b), Moore (1978), Tefft and Simeonsson (1979), and Wertlieb and Budman (1979). Rather than provide a comprehensive review of these issues here, we present two examples which serve to illustrate the important concerns for the MHP in primary care settings. One problem involves the professional identity of the MHP, as he or she experiences it and as others perceive it. The second example relates to broader political and economic problems.

Barksy (1980) notes:

> [the] primary care movement is itself internally confused and conflicted. Each of the medical specialties contends for territorial hegemony, while other health professionals struggle for greater role definition. The organization of practices, the structure and desirability of teaching programs, and the schemes of financial reimbursement all remain unsettled [p. 229].

In their discusssion of role conflicts for health care psychologists, Wertlieb and Budman (1979) identify three dimensions along which identity confusion and resolution may affect the MHP in a primary care setting: "Tradition versus Innovation, Autonomy versus Interdependency, and Paradigm Congruence versus Clash." The first, Tradition versus Innovation, defines the extent to which the MHP emphasizes traditional mental health concepts or skills, in contrast to new roles and concepts generated for and from MHP-PCP collaboration. Autonomy versus Interdependency refers to the common problems of divided loyalties, split responsibilites, and fragmented support systems often characteristic of current health care delivery systems and almost inevitably part of multidisciplinary efforts. Indeed, the degree of autonomy or integration of the MHP with the PHP team is the subject of some controversy (Coleman & Patrick, 1978; Budman, 1981; Pincus, 1980; Shepherd, 1979). The third dimension, Paradigm Congruence versus Clash, addresses the extent to which there is a match or mismatch, a "goodness of fit," among the conceptual or philosophical orientations of primary care team members, including the MHP.

At the political and economic level, there are important controversies which influence MHPs in primary care settings. Public policy debates over the relative merits of health maintenance organizations, community mental health centers, and neighborhood health centers, within the established primary care priority, have significant implications for MHP roles. One concern in the debate over national health insurance is whether or how to include the MHP. Further, concern over which MHPs to include— psychiatrists, psychologists, social workers, or nurses—has rekindled interdisciplinary rivalries and professional turf battles. Funding, reimbursement, even professional survival appear at stake (O'Keefe & McCullough, 1979; Richman, Brown, & Hicks, 1979).

Despite these problems, there is a justifiable energy and purpose for a better articulation of the contributions of MHP to primary care. There is by now an almost orthodox commitment to the holistic and biopsychosocial perspectives, along with impressive bodies of research literature justifying such commitment. Though individual MHPs may be confronted with the problems of role identity or with political and economic obstacles, there appears to be growing definition, acceptance, and support for MHP participation in primary care. Whether or not this participation will be a positive contribution are political and empirical questions to be addressed by future debate and research efforts. Many others concerned with the delivery of health care services are encouraging movement beyond our currently primitive base, as a critical and necessary responsibility (Barksy, 1980; Enelow, 1981; Pardes, 1979; Van Dyke, Rice, Pallett, & Leigh, 1980; Wertlieb & Budman, 1981). Over 100 years ago Wynter (1875, cited by Shepherd, 1979) propounded:

> We are convinced that for the good of general medicine, this particular study of psychological medicine, dealing as it does with so many complex problems should be merged in the general routine of medical practice [p. 223].

References

Abram, H. S. Primary care and consultation-liaison psychiatry. *Journal of Nervous and Mental Disease,* 1977, 164, 301-304.

Alpert, J., & Charney, E. *The education of physicians for primary care.* DHEW Publication No. (HRA) 74-3113. Washington, DC: Government Printing Office, 1974.

American Psychological Association, Task Force on Health Research. Contribution of psychology to health research. *American Psychologist,* 1976, 31, 263-274.

Authier, J. The family life cycle seminars: An innovative health care psychology program. *Professional Psychology,* 1979, 10, 451-457.

Barksy, A. J. Defining psychiatry in primary care: Origins, opportunities, and obstacles. *Comprehensive Psychiatry,* 1980, 21, 221-232.

Bibace, R., & Walsh, M. Clinical developmental psychologists in family practice settings. *Professional Psychology,* 1979, 10, 441-450.

Bibring, G. L. Psychiatry and medical practice in a general hospital. *New England Journal of Medicine,* 1956, 254, 366-372.

Bott, E. A. Teaching psychology in the medical course. *Bulletin of the Association of American Medical Colleges,* 1928, 3, 289-304.

Brill, N. Q. Introduction to psychiatric liaison. In R. O. Pasnau (Ed.), *Consultation-liaison psychiatry.* New York: Grune and Stratton, 1975.

Budman, S. H. (Ed.). *Forms of brief psychotherapy.* New York: Guilford Press, 1981.

Carey, K., & Kogan, W. Exploration of factors influencing physician decisions to refer patients for mental health services. *Medical Care,* 1971, 9, 55-66.

Cobb, S. Social support as a moderation of life stress. *Psychosomatic Medicine,* 1976, 38, 300-314.

Cohen, F. Personality stress and the development of physical illness. In G. Cohen et al. (Eds.), *Health psychology*. San Francisco: Jossey-Bass, 1979.

Coleman, J., & Patrick, D. L. Psychiatry and general health care. *American Journal of Public Health*, 1978, 68, 451-457.

Cummings, N., & VandenBos, G. The general practice of psychology. *Professional Psychology*, 1979, 10, 430-440.

Eisenberg, L. Disease and illness. *Culture, Medicine and Psychiatry*, 1977, 1, 9-23. (a)

Eisenberg, L. The search for care. *Daedalus*, 1977, 106, 235-246. (b)

Enelow, A. J. Consultation-liaison psychiatry. In H. Kaplan, A. M. Freedman, & B. Sadock (Eds.), *Comprehensive textbook of psychiatry*. Baltimore, MD: Williams and Wilkins, 1981.

Engel, G. L. The need for a new medical model: A challenge for biomedicine. *Science*, 1977, 196, 129-136.

Engel, G. L. The clinical application of the biopsychosocial model. *American Journal of Psychiatry*, 1980, 137, 535-544.

Feldman, A. The family practitioner as psychiatrist. *American Journal of Psychiatry*, 1978, 135, 728-731.

Fink, P. J. Psychiatry and the primary care physician. In H. Kaplan, A. M. Freedman, & B. Sadock (Eds.), *Comprehensive textbook of psychiatry*. Baltimore, MD: Williams and Wilkins, 1981.

Freedman, A. M., & Sack, R. L. Contributions of psychiatry to primary care medicine. In A. M. Freedman, R. L. Sack, & P. A. Berger (Eds.), *Psychiatry for the primary care physician*. Baltimore, MD: Williams and Wilkins, 1979.

Freedman, A. M., Sack, R. L., & Berger, P. A. (Eds.). *Psychiatry for the primary care physician*. Baltimore, MD: Williams and Wilkins, 1979.

Goldberg, R. L., Haas, M. R., Eaton, J. W., & Grubbs, J. H. Psychiatry and the primary care physician. *Journal of the American Medical Association*, 1976, 236, 944-945.

Haggerty, R. J., Roghmann, K. J., & Pless, I. B. *Child health and the community*. New York: John Wiley, 1975.

Hankin, J. Literature review on management of emotionally disturbed patients in primary care settings. In *Mental health services in general health care, vol. 1*. Washington, DC: Institute of Medicine, National Academy of Sciences, 1979.

Hankin, J., & Oktay, J. *Mental disorder in primary medical care: An analytical review of the literature*. DHEW Publication No. (ADM) 78-661. Washington, DC: Government Printing Office, 1979.

Harrington, R. Balm for the worried well (interview). *Innovations*, 1978, Fall, 3-10.

Illich, I. *Medical nemesis: The expropriation of health*. New York: Pantheon, 1976.

Institute of Medicine. *A manpower policy for primary care*. Washington, DC: National Academy of Sciences, 1978.

Institute of Medicine. *Mental health services in general health care, vol. 1*. Washington, DC: National Academy of Sciences, 1979.

Jacobson, A. The role of the psychiatrist in primary care settings: Issues and problems. In *Mental health services in general health care, vol. 1*. Washington, DC: Institute of Medicine, National Academy of Sciences, 1979.

Kagan, J. The new marriage: Pediatrics and psychology. *American Journal of Diseases of Children*, 1965, 110, 272-278.

Kahana, R. S. Teaching medical psychology through psychiatric consultation. *Journal of Medical Education*, 1959, 34, 1003-1009.

Kaplan, H. Treatment of psychosomatic disorders. In H. Kaplan, A. M. Freedman, & B. Sadock (Eds.), *Comprehensive textbook of psychiatry*. Baltimore, MD: Williams and Wilkins, 1981.

Kline, N. S. Antidepressant medications: A more effective use by general practitioners, family physicians, internists, and others. *Journal of the American Medical Association*, 1974, 227, 1158-1160.

Krakowski, A. J. Consultation-liaison psychiatry: A psychosomatic service in the general hospital. In Z. J. Lipowski, D. R. Lipsitt, & P. C. Whybrow (Eds.), *Psychosomatic medicine: Current trends and clinical applications*. New York: Oxford University Press, 1977.

Lipowski, Z. J. Review of consultation psychiatry and psychosomatic medicine. I. General Principles. *Psychosomatic Medicine*, 1967, 29, 153-171. (a)

Lipowski, Z. J. Review of consultation psychiatry and psychosomatic medicine. II. Clinical aspects. *Psychosomatic Medicine*, 1967, 29, 201-224. (b)

Lipowski, Z. J. Consultation-liaison psychiatry: An overview. *American Journal of Psychiatry*, 1974, 131, 623-630.

Lipowski, Z. J. Consultation-liaison psychiatry: Past, present, and future. In R. O. Pasnau (Ed.), *Consultation-liaison psychiatry*. New York: Grune and Stratton, 1975.

Lipowski, Z. J. Psychiatric consultation: Concepts and controversies. *American Journal of Psychiatry*, 1977, 134, 523-528. (a)

Lipowski, Z. J. Psychosomatic medicine in the seventies: An overview. *American Journal of Psychiatry*, 1977, 134, 233-244. (b)

Martin, M. Psychiatry and medicine. In H. Kaplan, A. M. Freedman, & B. Sadock (Eds.), *Comprehensive textbook of psychiatry*. Baltimore, MD: Williams and Wilkins, 1980.

Matarazzo, J. D. Behavioral health and behavioral medicine: Frontiers for a new health psychology. *American Psychologist*, 1980, 35, 807-817.

Mechanic, D. *Future issues in health care: Social policy and the rationing of medical services*. New York: Free Press, 1979.

Meyer, E., & Mendelson, M. Psychiatric consultations with patients on medical and surgical wards: Patterns and processes. *Psychiatry*, 1961, 24, 197-220.

Millon, T., Green, L., & Meagher, R. The MBHI: A new inventory for the psychodiagnostician in medical settings. *Professional Psychology*, 1979, 10, 529-539.

Moore, G. L. The adult psychiatrist in the medical environment. *American Journal of Psychiatry*, 1978, 135, 413-419.

Mumford, E., Schlesinger, H., & Glass, G. V. Problems of analyzing the cost offset of including a mental health component in primary care. In *Mental health services in general health care, vol. 1*. Washington, DC: Institute of Medicine, National Academy of Sciences, 1979.

Nason, F., & Delbanco, T. L. Soft services: A major cost-effective component of primary medical care. *Social Work in Health Care*, 1976, 1, 297-308.

O'Keefe, A. M., & McCullough, S. J. Physician domination in the health care industry: The pursuit of antitrust redress. *Professional Psychology*, 1979, 10, 605-618.

Oken, D., & Fink, P. J. General psychiatry: A primary-care specialty. *Journal of the American Medical Association*, 1976, 235, 1973-1974.

Olbrisch, M. Psychotherapeutic interventions in physical health. *American Psychologist*, 1977, 32, 761-777.

Pardes, H. The provision of mental health services in primary care settings. In *Mental health services in general health care, vol. 1*. Washington, DC: Institute of Medicine, National Academy of Sciences, 1979.

Pelletier, K. R. (Ed.). *Holistic medicine: From pathology to optimum health*. New York: Dell, 1979.

Pincus, H. Linking general health and mental health systems of care: Conceptual models of implementation. American Journal of Psychiatry, 1980, 137, 315-320.

Rachman, S. J., & Philips, C. Psychology of behavioral medicine. New Haven, CT: Cambridge University Press, 1980.

Regier, D. A., Goldberg, I. D., & Taube, C. A. The de facto U.S. mental health services system. Archives of General Psychiatry, 1978, 35, 685-693.

Richman, A., Brown, M., & Hicks, V. Reimbursement for mental health services in primary care settings. In Mental health services in general health care, vol. 1. Washington, DC: Institute of Medicine, National Academy of Sciences, 1979.

Rittelmeyer, L. F., & Flynn, W. E. Psychiatric consultation in an HMO: a model for education in primary care. American Journal of Psychiatry, 1978, 135, 1089-1092.

Rogers, D. E. The challenge of primary care. Daedalus, 1977, 106, 81-103.

Rosen, G. M., Geyman, J. P., & Layton, R. H. (Eds.). Behavioral science in family practice. New York: Appleton-Century-Crofts, 1980.

Schlesinger, H. J., Mumford, E., & Glass, G. V. The effects of psychological intervention on recovery from surgery. In F. Guerra & J. A. Aldrete (Eds.), Emotional responses to anesthesia and surgery. New York: Grune and Stratton, 1981.

Schofield, W. The role of psychology in the delivery of health services. American Psychologist, 1969, 24, 565-584.

Schofield, W. Clinical psychologists as health professionals. In G. Stone, F. Cohen, & N. Adler (Eds.), Health psychology: A handbook. San Francisco: Jossey-Bass, 1979.

Schwartz, G. E., & Weiss, S. On What is behavioral medicine? Psychosomatic Medicine, 1977, 39, 377-381.

Shepherd, M. Plenary presentation, April 3, 1979: Mental health as an integrant of primary care. In Mental health services in general health care, vol. 1. Washington, DC: Institute of Medicine, National Academy of Sciences, 1979.

Smilkstein, G. A model for applying behavioral science to family practice. In G. M. Rosen, J. P. Geyman, & R. H. Layton (Eds.), Behavioral science in family practice. New York: Appleton-Century-Crofts, 1980.

Stachnik, T. J. Priorities for psychology in medical education and health care delivery. American Psychologist, 1980, 35, 8-15.

Stone, G. C., Cohen, F., & Adler, N. (Eds.). Health psychology: A handbook. San Francisco: Jossey-Bass, 1979.

Tefft, B., & Simeonsson, R. Psychology and the creation of health care settings. Professional Psychology, 1979, 10, 558-570.

Van Dyke, C., Rice, D., Pallett, P., & Leigh, H. Psychiatric consultation: Compliance and level of satisfaction with recommendations. Psychotherapy and Psychosomatics, 1980, 33, 14-24.

Watson, J. B. Content of a course in psychology for medical students. Journal of the American Medical Association, 1912, 58, 916-918.

Wertlieb, D. A preventive health paradigm for health care psychologists. Professional Psychology, 1979, 10, 548-557.

Wertlieb, D., & Budman, S. H. Dimensions of role conflict for the health care psychologist. Professional Psychology, 1979, 10, 640-644.

Wertlieb, D., & Budman, S. H. The health-mental health linkage: Mandates and challenges for program evaluation research. In G. Stahler and W. Tash (Eds.), Innovative approaches to mental health evaluation. New York: Academic Press, 1981.

West, N. D. Psychiatry in primary care medicine. Chicago: Year Book Medical Publishers, 1979.

Wexler, M. The behavioral sciences in medical education. *American Psychologist*, 1976, 31, 275-283.

Wildavsky, A. Doing better and feeling worse: The political pathology of health policy. *Daedalus*, 1977, 106, 105-123.

Wright, L. The pediatric psychologist: A role model. *American Psychologist*, 1967, 22, 323-325.

Wright, L. Health care psychology: Prospects for the well-being of children. *American Psychologist*, 1979, 34, 1001-1006.

Wynter, A. The role of the general practitioner. In *The borderlands of insanity*. London: Hardwicke, 1875.

Zuckerman, B., Carper, J., & Alpert, J. Mental health training for pediatricians. *Journal of Clinical Child Psychology*, 1978, 7, 43-46.

8

Psychological Services and Health Enhancement

A Corporate Model

James S. J. Manuso

*The Equitable Life Assurance Society
of the United States, New York*

Introduction

Increasingly, corporations are seeing themselves in the role of health care service providers for their employees. With this new perspective comes the naivete that gives rise to radical experiments in the design and implementation of health care systems. Unencumbered by a stale, stodgy, and expensive network of traditional health care provision hierarchies and systems, modern corporations may well be in a position to revolutionize cost-controlled, health enhancement, and disease prevention programs for employees. The traditional boundaries on the professional focus of the psychologist are unknown to corporate management and are therefore largely nonexistent in corporate work.

Large organizations, in an effort to maximize their incrementally decreasing return on investments in human resources, have recognized their role as a stressor. Because large organizations are dynamic, the stressors they generate are frequent, intense, sustained, creating an environment conducive to the development of stress-related disorders and other degenerative diseases. In turn, such disorders bring about significant deficits in the application of employees' social, intellectual, and learned skills, which are particularly important in organizational life. Moreover, these deficits are communicable in a social environment, bringing about measurable productivity declines. Since this means a measurable net loss to the organization, the selfishly altruistic need to correct the problem in a cost-effective manner, consistent with sound business practice, becomes paramount. This mandate is fortunate for the mental health industry, which needs to become more cost-effective and preventive in its applications.

There are other social, legal, and economic reasons for a growing cottage industry of corporate mental health policies and programs at this time in our history. American society has become increasingly complex, demanding rapid change, both interpersonally and institutionally. Previously avoidable confrontations with the full emancipation of women and minorities, with job changes, new sex roles, social alienation, divorce, relocation, greater competition, and new technologies and management systems are no longer avoidable. It should come as no surprise that the President's Commission on Mental Health (Manuso, 1978) suggests that 25 percent of all Americans are suffering severe emotional stress, that the majority of Americans are dying from the stress-related disorders, primarily through heart attack and associated hypertension and coronary artery disease, and that one-third to one-half of all general practice patients—including those seen in corporate medical departments—are presenting with stress-related problems. Americans, feeling more health-conscious and seeking a higher quality of life, are recognizing the importance of assisted behavioral change. Psychological health care is becoming less of a stigma and more widely accepted; people feel they need not be "sick" in order to get better and are taking more preventive approaches to personal health care. Employees, corporations, and unions are all being educated as to the benefits of preventive mental health measures. A "new breed" of employees, younger and more politically and socially sensitive, are insisting on corporate social responsibility and its associated services.

From a legal perspective, with the advent of affirmative action and equal employment opportunity, comes the corporation's responsibilities for ensuring the success and development of women, minorities, and the disabled. Thus, the vast problems of inner-city minorities, who have historically received the least of the worst mental health care, become the problems of the employing corporation. People cannot be fired, nor can hiring be denied, for health-related problems which affect an employee's overall performance. The maintenance of confidentiality with respect to employee health records has encouraged employees to make use of corporate mental health programs. Furthermore, corporations continue to eschew governmental mandate, preferring to act before being acted upon.

From a purely economic perspective, profit-minded corporations can no longer afford to close their eyes to the stress-related genesis of costly employee lateness and absenteeism, poor decisions, terminations, dissension in work groups, lost sales, lowered worker morale, overtime costs, disciplinary actions, grievances, and the like. Thus, the corporate bill for our nation's health care costs and employee benefits (now one-third of salary and increasing) is emerging more and more on the balance sheet. On the services end, there are more mental health practitioners available, practitioners trained in interventions that are typically short in duration, making use of drugs and new more effective and less expensive technologies. Finally, because most corporations already sponsor employee medical departments, it becomes a relatively inexpensive task to integrate a mental health program into an already existing health service.

At its home office, Equitable Life Assurance Society of the United States employs approximately 7000 people. Of these 1600 are officers and upper-level managers, the majority of whom are white males. Most of the 70 percent of women employed hold lower-level jobs, primarily of a clerical nature, as do minorities. Associated with Equitable's commitment to hire and train inner-city youths are many of the problems of an urban population—below-average educational backgrounds, substance abuse, a lack of "institutional sophistication," resistance to authority, and poor coping skills. The Equitable organization is characterized by hierarchical control, exhibiting an increasingly decentralized pyramidal structure within each of four operating complexes and for the organization as a whole. It is a nonunionized corporation, which places special demands on management to see that employee satisfaction, in terms of salary benefits, help on personal problems, career growth, good working conditions, and the like, is maintained at a high level. Historically, Equitable has encouraged employee dependency, with the result that employee length of services is high. Using Equitable as an example, a variety of issues and preventive mental health policies and programs will be examined in this chapter.

Corporate Stressors
and Populations at Risk

The major stressor in corporate life is the single massive organizational change, the prototype of which is job abolishment. In connection with the recent Three Mile Island problem, the major concern of the employees was not the fear of radiation exposure, but the possibility of shutdown and loss of jobs. Loss of one's job involves a loss of self-esteem, resulting in suppressed anger and the potential for depression. When a whole group of jobs are abolished, it is highly stressful for those left behind. There is uncertainty, guilt, anger, and a feeling of helplessness. There is also a question of trust and uncertainty regarding the organization. No organization is immune.

There are ten major occupational stressors:

- work overload or work stagnation—too much or too little to do;

- ambiguity or rigidity in relation to one's tasks;

- extreme role conflict or little conflict—is the fit right with regard to the job?;

- extreme amounts of responsibility, particularly for people;

- negative competition—"your job stinks, but mine is very good"—or no competition;

- constant change and daily variability, or deadening stability;

- ongoing contact with stress carriers, i.e., workaholics, highly anxious individuals, indecisive individuals or depressed people who influence others' stress levels—or at the other extreme, social isolation;

- an organizational climate which encourages containment of emotional reactions and ego identification with the organization (which can lead to suppressed hostility and stress-related disorders);

- a poor interaction of career opportunity with management style; and, finally,

- many things related to corporate office work—meetings, daily deadlines, talking with the boss, writing memos, business lunches, presentations to management, late appointments.

Taken alone, these stressors may be insignificant, but on a continuous basis they are critical. Women and minorities are particularly affected because they are new to corporate life and must do more coping and adapting.

Any corporate employee finds him or herself in a "management sandwich," though this is especially true of the middle manager, who, automation experts tell us, may be an endangered species. As automated systems replace purveyors and managers of the information flow, old jobs will die and new ones will be developed. In addition, the baby boom of the late 1940s and early 1950s is beginning to crowd its way into corporate America, demanding fast-track, middle-management jobs. This cohort is well-educated and fully embued with the psychology of entitlement, which will make for heightened competition and disappointment.

It is clear that the stressors reviewed in this section will have an impact on the health profiles of corporate employees at all levels. The mental health professional working in a corporate health department must be aware of them and must plan for interventions which will impact on the disorders resulting from these conditions, on an individual, group, and organization-wide basis. Coordination with medical and allied health professional staffs is necessary if any employee health programs are to succeed.

Coordinating Medical and Psychological Services in the Emotional Health Program

There are three distinct phases in the development of Equitable's Emotional Health Program. It began in 1956 with the advent of an alcoholism program. It was staffed with a half-time physician, who later became the chairman of the National Council on Alcoholism, and one recovered alcoholic who functioned as a counselor. This program was expanded in 1969 to include other substance abusers, primarily narcotics addicts. The guiding policy has remained unchanged; namely, that substance abuse per se is a medical and psychological problem requiring appropriate treatment and administrative monitoring. Once identified by management, a substance abusing employee is referred to a program staff member who decides upon the nature of treatment indicated by the medical and psychological extent of substance abuse. The employee is then offered the opportunity to undertake treatment or to face the administrative consequences of his or her behavior. The overwhelming majority of identified substance abusers choose treatment and are followed up periodically by Emotional Health Program personnel. As with all health center transactions, visits are completely confidential. Thus, the early phase program began as primarily a reconnaissance and referral service, tending not to treat employees in-house. This is usually referred to as a "job-jeopardy" program, for obvious reasons.

The social and economic successes of the substance abuse program and the realities of emotional problems among employees prompted further commitment to the troubled employee. In 1972, the groundwork for the current Emotional Health Program was initiated. A group of psychologist-consultants was contracted to study and report upon the problem of troubled employees, to offer short-term treatment and referrals, and to train certain personnel and medical department employees in the recognition and handling of the troubled employee. The overwhelmingly positive response of management and employees to the presence of an effective and confidential psychological service led to the third, present-day phase of the Emotional Health Program (EHP).

An Equitable, it is corporate policy to provide a program of health care for employees during the working day and to assist management in handling problems in which the physical or emotional well-being of an employee may be involved. The overall employee health program is the responsibility of the Employee Health Services Department at the New York home office. The Emotional Health Program of the Employee Health Services Department is dedicated to the detection, prevention, education, treatment, referral, and follow-up of troubled employees. All services are completely confidential, free of charge, and on company time. Employee emotional health problems are recognized as treatable and do not jeopardize one's job.

The EHP is physically housed in the Employee Health Services Department, thereby enabling the delivery of multimodality (psychological and medical) services. Company physicians and nurses work closely with Emotional Health Program staff; the latter varies in size from one practitioner for every 2000 employees during times of "business as usual" to one for every 1000 employees during times of major organizational change. Today, the EHP is staffed with a psychologist, a psychiatrist, and two psychology interns. Liaisons are maintained with outside mental health practitioners, universities, hospitals, and related institutions.

The EHP offers a variety of optional and confidential services to employees, including short-term psychological treatment (i.e., 10 sessions or less) for anxiety and depression, the stress-related disorders, phobias, sexual dysfunction, and related nonpsychotic problems. Two major modalities are used, conventional insight-oriented and cognitive-behavioral psychotherapy, and the Stress Management Training Program. This latter mode is industry's first in-house biofeedback laboratory, founded at Equitable in 1975, wherein clients are neuromuscularly reeducated, or taught to achieve and maintain low levels of psychological and physical arousal in the face of stressors. Psychological diagnostic testing is offered, but not for purposes of employee selection. The Substance Abuse Program for self-referred or otherwise identified alcoholic and other drug abusers remains unchanged from the original program: Clients are offered the option of treatment with follow-up or facing the administrative consequences of their drug-induced behavior. The overwhelming majority of identified substance abusers continue to choose treatment.

EHP staff members are always on immediate call for acute crisis situations involving, for example, suicidal or homicidal threats, psychotic episodes, and aggressive behavior. The Managerial Training Program offers presentations to managers and supervisors regarding the recognition, proper handling, and appropriate referral of troubled employees. Advisory and consultative services are available to management for assistance in solving social and psychological problems encountered in their work. For example, the program has been consulted regarding the issues of relocation, job abolishment, decentralization, employee morale, and even environmental design. Employees requiring or requesting longer-term or highly specialized care are referred to the proper outside agency, institution, or practitioner. Follow-up is always a necessary part of referral out. In order to maximize the quality of health care offered to employees, liaisons are maintained with major teaching and research institutions in major American cities. Whenever a common problem, such as job abolishment, is shared by a large number of employees, some form of group intervention may be undertaken (Manuso, 1977b).

The experience of the Emotional Health Program shows that the vast majority of troubled employees do not present job-related problems but personal, situational, or interpersonal problems. In decreasing order of frequency, the problems seen are anxiety disorders (25 percent); depression (20 percent); stress-related disorders, including headache, generalized tension, myalgia, etc. (15 percent); substance abuse (15 percent); situational problems such as a death in the family or financial dilemmas (10 percent); and all others (15 percent). Although males and females use the services of the program in equal proportions, males tend to require more sessions of treatment than do females. This difference appears to occur because males tend to minimize or ignore the warning signals of emotional problems, whereas women respond quickly to emotional disequilibrium and seek out the proper care sooner, thereby arresting further symptoms development. The program's experience demonstrates that the group reporting the most severe problems is composed of white or Hispanic males ages 20 to 39, married, with five or more years of service, working in presupervisory and premanagerial jobs. It is here, during the take-off phase for one's family and career lives, the occupational and other stressors have their greatest additive impact.

With respect to the number of employees utilizing the program, in 1978 five staff saw 500 individuals in approximately 2500 visits. This utilization represented approximately 13 percent of the home office employee population. The group was comprised of 58 percent females and 42 males. A recent study indicated that 60 percent of all employees who received mental health services stated that these services were very helpful in terms of positive changes in the initial problem, their life in general, attendance, job performance, and job satisfaction. Thirty percent said that the services were somewhat helpful, 8 percent said they were not helpful, and 2 percent did not respond. Therefore, 90 percent of EHP services were self-reported to be concretely helpful. Thus, it has been demonstrated that employees suffering mental health problems may be effectively treated at their work site. This approach has a potential for primary prevention and health enhancement.

Program Evolution

Generally, emotional health programs such as the one at Equitable tend to evolve in specific directions over time. There is a tendency to move from a curative (that is, disability-oriented) stance to one of prevention and health enhancement. There is a movement away from addressing only the most severe problems with gross consequences to recognizing the importance of working with milder problems that nonetheless create significant hidden costs. Over time there is a tendency to refer out less and offer more in-house, short-term treatment. Correspondingly, staff size increases and service patterns shift. From a one-on-one orientation in intervention, there develops a willingness to work with groups of employees. As programs grow, they become more powerful in the host institution, establishing more liaisons with external resources, particularly with universities. Internship programs develop and research begins to emanate from the program. There develops an access to senior management, and program roles expand. As a critical mass of practitioners is achieved, more aggressive marketing of the program to employees takes place. Although more passive counseling strategies typically characterize the beginning program, a mature program begins to offer active interventions based on behavior modification approaches. The staff, originally paraprofessionals to a great extent, are replaced with mental health professionals. The program, originally cloistered and silent in the corporation, becomes more visible and communicative; there are more interactions and coordinations with other departments in the organization and a greater willingness to address the press, usually through film productions and radio programs. The original practitioner evolves into an administrator and manager as the staff size increases. The program, providing it has proven its worth in the competitive corporate arena and thereby earned the respect of the corporate system, enjoys a "free agent" status in the organization and is trusted by the corporation.

A Preventive Stress Management Training Program for Employees

Although certainly there are coordinating efforts between physicians, other health professionals, and psychologists in the employee counseling function, this coordination becomes a fuller, multimodal service when psychologists begin to address health areas previously considered the domain of medicine—that is, psychophysiological disorders, behavioral practices conducive to the development of the iatrogenic illnesses, and health education. This section will describe the Stress Management Training Program (SMTP), which often requires the coordination of physicians, physiotherapists, and psychologists.

It is of note that the SMTP, a biofeedback-based, relaxation and coping skills acquisition program, found its genesis in the treatment of a 60-year-old female with a six-year history of chronic exzematous dermatitis of the hands (Manuso, 1977a). A powerful corporate physician, frustrated by the failures of medicine in her case and skeptical of biofeedback treatment, referred her to the EHP. The patient learned handwarming, remitted in her symptoms, and remained symptom-free at the six-month follow-up. Good timing for the beginning of an important program!

Equitable's Stress Management Training Program is intended to assist people with stress-related disorders and uses muscle tension and temperature biofeedback. The program is intended to identify and train in the practice of stress-management techniques those employees who evidence some suffering from the symptoms of stress overloads. This section will describe recently completed research (Manuso, 1980) on the Stress Management Training Program.

There are four stages of the SMPT. The first is a two-week intake phase, wherein the employee with a chronic stress-related disorder refers him or herself or is referred by a physician in the health center. Common presenting problems are tension or vascular headache, generalized anxiety, or myalgia. In some instances, hypertension, pain, dermatitis, general intestinal dysfunctions, and the like are treated. Screening is conducted via a medical neurological and psychological evaluation, in which a level of symptom activity (a composite of intensity and frequency of the symptom) must be found to be at least in the moderate to severe range. Finally, the patient must be "motivated" for treatment. Members of the screening team confer before referring an employee in order to ensure that all possible treatment complications and other health problems are appropriately addressed. We must not forget that Gershwin died of a brain tumor while undergoing psychoanalysis administered by a physician! Our psychological interventions are no more sacrosanct than medical ones and should be regularly challenged and scrutinized.

In the second, baseline phase, also lasting two weeks, the employee comes to the Biofeedback Laboratory once a week, where forehead tension and hand temperature baseline measures are taken during a "stress state" and a "relaxed state." In the baseline phase employees also fill out two weeks of a daily log of symptom activity and behavior. This instrument also indicates their symptoms' interference with their functioning in the world.

The third phase constitutes treatment lasting five weeks. During this time individuals come to the Biofeedback Lab for deep relaxation training two to three times weekly. They receive primarily forehead muscle tension feedback with both audio and visual components in the first week. In subsequent weeks, feedback is primarily audio. Each laboratory session lasts approximately 20 minutes with, ten one minute trials measured for the subjects. There is a postsession questionnaire inquiring as to the nature of the employee's twilight state mentation, interfering thought processes (which typically refer back to a person's daily work problems), their physical sensations during the session, and what they were doing to achieve relaxation.

To assist employees in their development of stress awareness and control, they receive a cassette relaxation program (Budzynski, 1975; Manuso, 1975), an article on biofeedback training (Green, 1977), a list of self-hypnotic, autogenic phrases (Cyborg Corporation, 1974), and verbal instructions for the twice-daily practice of deep relaxation in periods lasting from five to fifteen minutes. Employees are also taught a series of behavior modification, isometric, and breathing exercises in order to enhance their learning and application of the antistress response. Toward the end of treatment, they are weaned from the biofeedback machinery and from dependency on feedback. This is accomplished by initially interspersing trials of feedback, no feedback, and, ultimately, a complete series of no feedback sessions. For three months immediately following treatment no contact whatsoever is made with employees. They do not fill out the daily log and are given no special instructions other than to continue practicing what they have learned.

In the fourth and final phase, follow-up, lasting two weeks, baseline measurements are again taken, employees fill out the daily log and are medically and psychologically evaluated. Subsequent to the first three-month follow up, there are six-month and annual follow-ups.

Evaluation Results

The results of research on 30 individuals, fifteen with headaches and fifteen with anxiety, who participated in this program from intake to first follow-up show that they learned to decrease the absolute value of their forehead tension levels by approximately 50 percent and that the within-session variation or variability of such tension decreased by approximately 60 percent. Thus, their tension levels were at a lower level and were more consistent. Symptom activity decreased from the high moderate level to the low range. The interference of symptoms with ongoing activities decreased from 9 percent per hour to 1.5 percent per hour and, at work, from approximately 18 to 4 percent. The interference of symptoms at work is considerably higher than that in general, before-and-after treatment, because most of the stressors having the greatest impact in bringing about symptoms relate to work environments. Weekly medication intake decreased from seven to two pills per week ("pills" may be Fiorinal or Percodan for headache patients and Valium or Librium for anxiety patients). Monthly visits to the health center for stress-related and other symptoms also decreased, from two to less than one-half visit per month following treatment. Twilight state mental imagery reported during deep relaxation increased from none per session at baseline to approximately .6—nearly one image per session for all persons—at follow-up. The interfering thoughts that were reported during deep relaxation decreased from approximately three to slightly less than one per session at follow-up. Again, most of the interfering thought content related to the work environment. Finally, the number of physical sensations of relaxation, or "proprioceptive awareness," that people developed in the course of training increased from .22 per session at the outset to approximately 2.33 at follow-up.

Analysis of variance over all phases of the program showed that there were no significant differences between headache and anxiety cases on all measures but the number of interfering thoughts and twilight state images reported, thereby suggesting that a unitary dimension of dysfunction is shared by both of these stress-related disorders. It appears the anxiety cases, who were much more prone to experiencing interfering thought patterns, had more difficulty in relaxing to the point where twilight state mental imagery would begin to occur.

Program Costs

The *additional* weekly pretreatment costs to the corporation of employing one person (average salary equals $270.00) with chronic headache or anxiety amounted to $70. This cost derived from three major categories: first, visits to the health center; second, the interference of one's symptoms with his or her capacity to work; and third, "meta-interference," or the effect of one person's anxiety on a co-worker, a boss, and a subordinate. This represents the "stress carrier" potential of employees suffering from the chronic stress-related disorders. Thus, the total additional pretreatment costs to the corporation of employing individuals with stress-related disorders are not, as may have been suspected, related to lateness and absenteeism. The costs are hidden. The employees experiencing stress-related disorders typically work very hard, are not late, or put in extra hours, the effectiveness of their time is less than what it could be in the absence of interfering symptoms.

After treatment, the additional costs for employees with stress-related symptoms dropped dramatically to $15.00 per employee per week. Cumulative cost-benefit ratios demonstrate that for every dollar invested in such a program there is a $5.52 return on that investment per employee per year. Also on the financial side are the incidental observations that unchecked stress difficulties predispose employees to a higher-than-average likelihood of being terminated, and that employees suffering stress symptoms who complete the program are more likely to advance their careers in the corporation at rates higher than could the average employee.

It is evident that the Stress Management Training Program is a preventive and health-enhancing effort consistent with corporate objectives and individual health care concerns. For the corporation, offering stress management enhances productivity and decreases medical costs while decreasing the number of stress carriers, which would otherwise cause a diffusion of stress throughout the delicate social network of the corporation. For the individual employee, effective stress management frees time and enhances alertness, composure, and relaxation in the absence of interfering symptoms. Both employer and employee gain.

From Stress Management to Wellness

It should come as no surprise that the executive-corporate community, imbued with the need to control, is quick to endorse self-regulated programs for health enhancement, especially when the cost-benefit picture is favorable. In fact, executives' health profiles have always been among the best of all occupations (Warshaw, 1979), pointing up the sense of commitment modern corporations have expressed for their top people. It was in this spirit that the successes of the biofeedback-based SMTP prompted the development of a group-administered stress management training program for asymptomatic employees at Equitable Life.

The primary objective of the group-administered stress management training program was to train groups of twelve management employees in the core skills of appropriate stress management, including physiological, psychological, sociopsychological, and managerial techniques which would enhance their capacity to adapt to change and to an array of corporate and other stressors. This program was designed as a self-health program with the aim of enhancing health and promoting wellness. It relies completely on an individual's motivation to maintain his or her health profile and to create healthy habits where there were unhealthy ones.

In the course of two meetings of approximately four hours each, twelve individuals are taught the following seven core techniques of stress management: the quieting response (Stroebel, 1978), a method of deep relaxation (Budzynski, 1975), assertiveness, psychological coping strategies (including stress-inoculation and systematic desensitization), stretching and isometric exercises, proper dietary and nutritional practices, and a series of behavioral techniques for changing habits. The training staff consists of five professionals: three psychologists, one physician, and one physiotherapist.

The program proceeds sequentially across two weeks and then breaks for three months, with one two-hour follow-up meeting at the end of the three-month period. The program is broken down into five basic components, beginning with a presession, assessment phase. During this phase, participants are sent a health hazard appraisal which assesses their health profile and risk factors. They are also sent a number of blank daily logs, along with instructions for completing them, a modified symptom check list, an assertiveness inventory, a Type A-Type B scale, and a social readjustment rating scale (Holmes & Rahe, 1967). These instruments attract the participants' interest before the program and engage them in ongoing self-assessment procedure before it begins.

During the introductory and second sessions, participants are taught the seven core techniques which were outlined earlier. The program employs a variety of audiovisual, didactic, and interactive training sequences in order to accomplish its goals. Program participants are expected to complete a variety of "homework" assignments relating to their health profiles and their ways of coping with stressor situations. They are expected to practice the techniques which they are taught in order for these to have any significance in their lives. Basic experience has shown that approximately 75 percent of the participants do follow through with what has been taught (Manuso, in press).

Two months and two weeks after the second session, participants are sent another packet of materials containing daily logs and other instructions to begin self-assessment once again. In the final, follow-up session, all of the techniques are reviewed, and participants discuss their experiences in employing them. Participants assess their stress response and then begin to modify it. They also learn how to manage themselves in difficult, emotionally charged social situations, those which typically give rise to the stress response.

The ease with which the medical, physiotherapy, and psychology personnel relate to one another in presenting this program is quite remarkable. Continuity is maintained, and participants—including those who are critical at the outset—ultimately integrate one or more of the techniques into their daily practice.

Resulting from the observation that there is a series of specific techniques which can be taught in a stress management program, the author proceeded to develop an eight-hour, nonmediated, audiovisual package in stress management (Manuso, 1980). This training package, resulting from the efforts of seven psychologists and five physicians, represents the state of the art of stress management. The package includes a facilitator's guide, a film section, a series of audiotapes, and participants' self-assessment instruments and workbooks. The workbooks cover a review of the stress response and risk factors, personality types and their stress-proneness, the quieting response, diet and nutrition, substance abuse factors, physical exercise, self-monitoring techniques, psychological stress and irrational beliefs, stress inoculation, self-regulation techniques such as imaging and changing habits and beliefs, assertiveness training, recognizing and managing occupational stressors, developing support systems, and signing contingency contracts for change. The program also includes an audiotape with two relaxation exercises. This package is currently being field-tested, both in its self-mediated and professionally-mediated forms, in order to assess the actual behavior change it may or may not produce. The field test also compares a one-day administration method with a six-week administration method.

A natural offspring of stress management is the professionally mediated wellness program. Only recently have large organizations, such as the United States Center for Disease Control, Johnson and Johnson, and the Control Data Corporation, gone into the wellness business for their employees and for those of other corporations. In these instances, holistic medicine (Pelletier, 1979), stress management (Manuso, 1980), meditation (Benson, 1976), exercise (Cooper, 1970), and dietary self-management (Pritikin, 1979) strategies are combined with cognitive-behavioral methods (Meichenbaum, 1977) to produce group health behavior change. It is far too early to tell what real maintenance effects these programs will have, but early evidence, such as the data from the Stanford Pre-Community Study (Maccoby, Farguar, Wood, & Alexander, 1977), suggests that the impact may be very significant.

Equitable has developed a wellness program which not only relies on educational strategies and group administration but also makes use of individual "wellness practitioners." In its pilot effort in Charlotte, North Carolina, Equitable is field-testing this important program. Figure 8.1 is a schematic representation of the Equitable Health Management Program.

Employees are first screened for the data necessary for input to the health hazard appraisal. A health educator then assists employees in interpreting their health hazard appraisal and other assessment instruments with the aim of prioritizing specific behaviors for change. The employee is then referred to an intervention expert based on the life risk behavior representing the greatest risk or the one which the employee feels he or she can best work on. Throughout the course of this process there are monthly meetings chaired by one of the intervention experts wherein a health-related topic is discussed. In addition, there are close-ended support groups, lasting six weeks each, covering the topics of stress, exercise, diet, and nutrition.

Once the intervention experts such as nutritionists, physiologists, psychologists, or physicians, meet with the employee, the expert and the employee agree upon a health behavior goal and a time frame. Finally, the intervention takes place and follow-up occurs. If the employee reaches the health goal, he or she receives a corporate-donated reward, such as additional time off, the freedom to come into work later than the norm, special recognition luncheons, or others. Throughout this program, confidentiality is maintained, yet the employee is given a certificate of achievement of a health goal which is then presented to his or her manager who must then offer the reward. The program will continue on an ongoing basis for at least five years in order for Equitable to assess the behavioral, economic, and other impacts of this program.

Wellness programs such as this pilot program at Equitable will offer further opportunities for behavioral scientists to work closely with a variety of health professionals in the provision of a new array of services to employees of the future. Unlike other arenas of health care, prevention and health enhancement strategies appear to offer the opportunity for a unusual, co-equal status among the professionals involved in the program. The new field of behavioral medicine is permeating industry just as it is being recognized in academia. The outcome can only be beneficial for the American population.

Other Programs

A variety of other programs require the appropriate coordination of medical and psychological services at Equitable. For example, there is a health evaluation program wherein a poorly performing or otherwise problematic employee may be referred for a health evaluation by his or her supervisor.

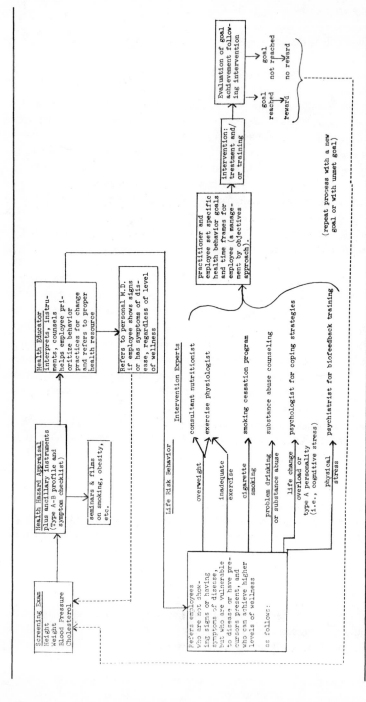

Figure 8.1: Flowchart of the Health Management Program

This request for health evaluation is reviewed conjointly by a psychologist, who then contact the supervisor for any additional information before meeting with the employee for an assessment meeting. The employee is then evaluated by the physician and the psychologist who then confer with each other before responding to the supervisor. Confidentiality is again maintained: The supervisor is notified only as to whether or not the employee represents a health-related problem, the employee's decision to treat or not to treat this problem, and any special considerations which might be involved. In the event that the employee does not present a health problem, the supervisor is instructed to proceed with appropriate administrative action. This instrument permits the medical and psychological staff to respond to real needs of supervisors and also assists employees in notifying them of the availability of appropriate services. In only a very few instances does the employee suffering, for example, a depression reject the opportunity for treatment.

During a period of job abolishment or "outplacement," employees are offered the opportunity to meet with a physician and a psychologist prior to leaving the organization (Manuso, 1977b). In addition to the availability of a professional outplacement counselor through a number of consulting firms, employees may take the opportunity to discuss with their physician or psychologist appropriate referrals elsewhere, their feelings regarding their separation from the organization, and any other issues of importance. Management has given Employee Health Services the mandate to extend the period of service delivery available to such employees approximately three to six months beyond their termination date.

For employees who are rehabilitating on the job, such as alcoholics, drug abusers, and the physically disabled, a physiotherapist, the medical staff, and the psychology staffs are available for consultation and follow-up. Occasionally, difficulties arise between the rehabilitating employee and the supervisor which may require mediation by a health professional. Depending upon the nature of the disability, the medical or psychology staffs will become involved, but only at the employee's request. In such instances, a semiadvocacy role is undertaken. In the future, it is hoped that the large numbers of "permanently" disabled Equitable employees may be assisted to return to work via the rehabilitation team intervention concept. This program has not yet been designed, but it is planned for the future.

The medical and psychology staffs are also active in the preretirement counseling program, wherein employees aged 55 or older are given a series of lectures and interactive opportunities concerning psychological, medical, legal, financial, geographical, and other issues related to retirement. The psychology staff also becomes involved in certain career counseling interventions, particularly when a psychological or medical function is uncovered. In some instances, psychology interns at Equitable are skilled in the areas of career counseling and are encouraged to offer such services through the Emotional Health Program.

Increasingly, as corporations recognize the critical role clinically trained psychologists can play, more opportunities will become available. Such opportunities previously may have been available only to the industrial-organizational psychologist whose area of expertise is not in the health services/clinical arena. As stated earlier, the possibility of sharing a co-equal status in coordinating psychological with medical services is great.

Staffing an Occupational Mental Health Program

Experience has shown that there are a number of critical factors in connection with the selection, training, and development of staff members for an employee counseling program (Manuso, 1980). It is of the utmost importance that staff members be skilled diagnosticians and practitioners of short-term and individual psychotherapy. The corporate environment requires that shorter-term, more directive interventions be used if such programs are to survive. As one executive once stated, "We are not in the business of mental health." This principle must be kept in mind at all times. Although many employees may be treated in the short-term model, others must be appropriately referred and followed up.

Staff members' educational background should be in clinical psychology, preferably at or beyond the doctoral level, with at least one program director who holds a Ph.D. Psychologists and clinical social workers holding the doctorate and suitably trained may also be considered for staff positions. Here again, the issue of professionalism arises. Corporations, typically naive in their perception of providers of mental health services, must be taught about the appropriateness of certain practitioners.

Ideally, staff members' prior work history should include experience in a corporate environment, in a medical setting, and, if necessary, with inner-city problems. The corporate environment is unique and needs to be understood by a mental health practitioner attempting to apply his or her skills in that environment. In addition, due to the importance of coordinating with the medical staffs, a background in a hospital or other medical setting is preferred. Finally, because many corporations are hiring inner-city employees who bring with them many inner-city problems, his area of understanding can be important. For the same reasons, staff should include appropriate female, minority, linguistic, and age-group representation, given the composition of the employee population to be addressed.

It appears that staff size should be on the order of one practitioner for every 2000 employees during times of "business as usual" and one for every 1000 employees during times of major organizational change, such as reorganization, regionalization, and job abolishment. Naturally, this ratio varies according to the industry involved and the specific practices of the program. Unfortunately, some programs continue to operate as a "pipeline" of feedback on employees to management; these program use very few practitioners for a large number of employees. This breach of confidentiality also jeopardizes the program and is a practice to be avoided if the corporation is serious in its desire to have an effective program.

Naturally, this new field will require skilled practitioners. As a result, Equitable has started the first occupational clinical psychology internship program in industry. The only other such program known to the author is the internship program at Wells Fargo Bank in San Francisco, California. These programs select promising doctoral candidates from leading institutions and offers them a full-time, one-year internship program with a unique focus on the problems characteristic of occupational clinical psychology. For example, an intern at the Equitable program will spend time on any one of the aforementioned programs, in addition to seeing individual clients.

The Equitable internship program offers group supervision through the program director, a psychologist, and through program's consulting psychiatrist. The program director also offers individual supervision to the interns. The interns are trained in cognitive-behavioral, short-term techniques, group administered approaches for health enhancement, and will have become involved in a variety of projects. Most recently, the interns have focused on the issues of psychological rehabilitation for disabled employees, evaluating agencies and individuals for a referral network, developing a handbook on the psychology of relocation, minor tranquilizer abuse among female employees, field-testing newly created health enhancement products, and a variety of other projects.

Started in 1976, the Equitable psychology internship program has trained approximately ten individuals, most of whom have decided to remain in one arm of occupational clinical psychology or another. It will not be much longer before other occupational clinical psychologists begin similar programs, within both universities and corporations.

Cost-Benefits

Of central concern to corporations is the cost-benefit picture of any health intervention they may choose to underwrite. For some time, the cost-benefits of health care interventions have been elusive. However, recently headway has been made in this important area.

Because alcoholism appears to have captured the attention of corporate health programs, in this arena some of the earliest cost-benefit research has been done. For example, Pritchett and Finley (1971) studied the costs of providing an alcoholism control program and the measurable costs of not providing such a program at a corporation of 1700 employees. The program costs amounted to $11,400, whereas the costs of not providing the program, to be found in lateness and absenteeism, poor decisions, terminations, early retirement, and so on, amounted to $100,650. Other research showed that for those General Motors employees seeking help for alcoholism, there was a 30 percent decrease in sickness benefits, a 56 percent decline in leaves of absence, a 63 percent decrease in disciplinary actions. A 78 percent decrease in the number of grievances filed, and an 82 percent decrease in job-related accidents (Stessin, 1977).

Research external to corporations on the financial impacts of psychotherapy has demonstrated the real benefits of this health care modality. For example, Reiss (1967) demonstrated that individuals seeking outpatient psychotherapy increased their work-related earnings during the course of treatment approximately 400 percent higher than did a control group of individuals in comparable occupations. Not only do people make more money as a result of psychotherapy, they also cost less from the perspective of a medical service provider or a third-party insurer. The work of Follette and Cummings (1967) has demonstrated that the utilization of outpatient *medical* services for a group of individuals receiving short-term psychotherapy decreased by 62 percent and their use of hospitalization decreased by 68 percent between the base year and the fifth year of the research. This decrease contrasted with the control group, whose medical care utilization maintained an escalating pattern over the full six years of the study. Recent research by Jameson et al. (1978) focused on the Blue Cross claims records of individuals utilizing outpatient psychiatric benefits over a four-year period. They found that overall medical/surgical utilization was reduced for that subgroup and that the average costs decreased by more than 50 percent per person.

Research on the cost-benefits of psychological interventions offered by employee counseling programs is relatively rare. However, research reported by the Kennecott Copper Company in Salt Lake City, Utah, indicates that their employee assistance program was responsible for cutting absenteeism in half and for contributing to a 55 percent reduction in hospital surgical medical costs (Egdahl & Walsh, 1980). Through the author's contacts within this emerging field, it is reported that interventions enjoy a return on investment on the order of 200 to 800 percent, depending upon the type of program, the setting, and the variables examined.

It is too early to tell the long-range effects these various forms of intervention will have. As mentioned earlier, the stress management and wellness programs, and those generally addressing any of the risk factors, are too early in their genesis to report reliable data. It is expected, however, that these preventive programs will demonstrate meaningful cost-benefits and will therefore proliferate.

Conclusion

Any corporation is a stressor to its employees. Corporations may be distinguished from one another, not in terms of the presence or absence of stressors, but in terms of their organizational response (or lack thereof) to the problem. It appears that the corporation's central objectives are to maximize profits in a competitive market and to thereby perpetuate itself, its growth, and its power through the management of employees, using rational and authoritarian organizational structures and systems. It is clear that corporations are not in the business of curative mental health. However, mental health promotion and preventive policies and programs are wholly consistent with corporate goals—and in fact enhance their achievement, as some corporations are learning.

The epoch of preventive health care, wellness, and self-regulation of behavior is truly beginning in corporate America. Increasingly, corporate employee health programs are serving as the lowest tier of preventive health service delivery. Government will no doubt encourage this development further, through financial and other incentives and, perhaps, through mandate. The tasks of developing and managing efficient, cost-effective preventive mental health programs will be met by the private sector—corporations must tame their creations for their own survival.

References

Benson, H. Your innate asset for combating stress. *Harvard Business Review,* 1976, July-August, 49-60.

Budzynski, T. CRP-1 cassette relaxation program. Boulder, CO: Biofeedback Systems, 1975.

Cooper, K. *The new aerobics.* New York: Evans & Co., 1970.

Cyborg Corporation. *Relaxation training procedure.* Boston, Massachusetts, 1974.

Egdahl, R., & Walsh, D. *Mental wellness programs for employees.* New York: Springer-Verlag, 1980.

Follette, W., & Cummings, N. Psychiatric services and medical utilization in a prepaid health plan setting: Kaiser Foundation Hospital, San Francisco. *Medical Care,* 1967, 5, 25-35.

Green, E. Biofeedback: What it is and how it can help you (interview). *U.S. News & World Report,* April 4, 1977, pp. 63-64.

Holmes, T., & Rahe, J. The social readjustment rating scale. *Journal of Psychosomatic Research,* 1967, 11, 213-218.

Jameson, J., Shuman, L., & Young, W. The effects of outpatient psychiatric utilization on the costs of providing third-party coverage. *Medical Care,* 1978, 16, 383-399.

Maccoby, N., Farquaar, J., Wood, P., & Alexander, J. Reducing the risk of cardiovascular disease: Effects of a community based campaign on knowledge and behavior. *Journal of Community Health,* 1977, 2, 100-114.

Manuso, J. A methodology for achieving low states of psychophysiological arousal. Cassette tape, 15 minutes, copyrighted.

Manuso, J. The issue of biofeedback-assisted hand warming training in the treatment of chronic exzematous dermatitis of the hands: A case study. *Journal of Behavior Therapy and Experimental Psychiatry,* 1977, 8, 445-446. (a)

Manuso, J. Coping with job abolishment. *Journal of Occupational Medicine,* 1977, 19, 598-602. (b)

Manuso, J. Testimony to the President's Commission on Mental Health, Panel on Costs and Financing. *Report of the President's Commission on Mental Health, vol. II,* appendix, p. 512. Washington, DC: Government Printing Office, 1978.

Manuso, J. *Manage your stress.* CRM Multimedia Module. New York: McGraw-Hill, 1980.

Manuso, J. Stress management training in a large corporation. *Biofeedback & Self-Regulation,* in press.

Meichenbaum, D. Cognitive behavior modification. New York: Plenum, 1977.

Pelletier, K. *Holistic medicine: From pathology to optimum health.* New York: Dell, 1979.

Pritchett, S., & Finley, L. Problem drinking and the risk management function. *Risk Management,* 1971, 18, 16-23.

Pritikin, H. *The Pritikin program for diet and exercise.* New York: Grosset & Dunlap, 1979.

Reiss, B. Changes in patient income concomitant with psychotherapy. *International Mental Health Research Newsletter,* 1967, 9, 1-4.

Stessin, L. When an employer insists. New York Times Business and Finance section, April 3, 1977.

Stroebel, D. *The quieting response.* BMA Cassette Series. New York.

Warshaw, L. *Managing stress.* Reading, MA: Addison-Wesley, 1979.

9

Community Mental Health and Organized Health Care Linkages

Edward Marks
University of South Florida
Anthony Broskowski
Northside Community Mental Health Center, Inc.
Tampa, Florida

The need for coordination between community mental health centers (CMHCs) and organized health care settings has recently received a great deal of recognition (President's Commission on Mental Health, 1978). Cooperative interorganizational arrangements are expected to improve the delivery of services, such as increasing service availability, comprehensiveness, and accessibility, as well as improving the quality of care provided to the public.

After a brief description of CMHCs and organized health care settings, this chapter will highlight the potential benefits and advantages of linking health and mental health service delivery. Specific mechanisms and models for such linkages will then be reviewed. Finally, we will summarize factors identified in the theoretical, case report, and research literature that may facilitate or inhibit the development and maintenance of effective linkages.

Community Mental Health Centers

As a result of dissatisfaction with existing mental health care, in 1955 Congress established a Joint Commission on Mental Illness and Health to

AUTHORS' NOTE: This chapter is based in part on work conducted under Contract No. 278-0030(OP) from the Primary Care Research Section of the Division of Biometry and Epidemiology of the National Institute of Mental Health, Dr. J. Burke, Contract Officer.

study mental illness and its treatment. Based on the commission's findings, Congress enacted legislation to establish community-based mental health centers. The Community Mental Health Centers Act of 1963 has since been amended several times as various government and private organizations have continued to evaluate and improve the status of mental health care in the United States (President's Commission on Mental Health, 1978).

As amended in 1975, the CMHC legislation (PL 94-63) mandated that federally funded CMHCs provide essential mental health services within a geographically defined "catchment area" of approximately 75,000 to 200,000 residents. The essential services are to include inpatient hospitalization (24-hour care); partial hospitalization; outpatient therapy; emergency services; screening, referral, aftercare, and transitional living facilities for chronic patients, as well as specialized services for high-risk populations of children, the elderly, and substance abusers. Also, consultation and education services, designed to assist other organizations and the community at large, are required.

Because the primary mission of the CMHC is to provide *comprehensive* care, such services are supposed to be readily available and accessible, and not hampered by geographic, cultural, linguistic, or economic barriers. Furthermore, CMHC services are to be well coordinated with the services of health and human service agencies. In this way, a CMHC does not have to provide all of the mandated services on its own, but can arrange for such services to be provided through affiliation agreements with other service providers.

Despite the requirements of PL 94-63, there have been continuing difficulties in providing accessible and comprehensive services to some of the highest-risk special populations, such as the poor and the elderly. A new law, PL 96-398, signed by President Carter on October 7, 1980, attempts to address some of these continuing deficiencies and shortcomings. The new Mental Health Systems Act focuses greater attention on high-risk groups, such as the chronic patient, the severely disturbed child, and the elderly. It also stresses a larger coordinative role at the level of state government while reducing the requirements for newly funded entities to be totally comprehensive before receiving any federal funds. Of specific interest to this chapter, Section 206 of the law provides for grants to "any public or non-profit private entity which provides mental health services . . . and has in effect an agreement of affiliation . . . with an entity which is a health care center." The affiliation agreement must describe the common geographical area to be served, provide for the employment of "at least one mental health professional to serve as a liaison," and provide assurances that the mental health entity will provide services to patients referred by the health center. The affiliation must also address "transportation . . . and other arrangements for affecting referral . . . of patients." The grant can cover the costs of the liaison staff, mental health services provided by other personnel, and consultation and inservice training to personnel of the health care center. A "health care center" is defined in this law to include "an outpatient facility operated in connection with a hospital, a primary care center, a community health center, a migrant health center, a clinic of the Indian Health Service, or skilled nursing home, an intermediate care facility, and an outpatient health care facility of a medical group practice, a public health department, or a health maintenance organization."

Organized Health Care Settings

The types of organized health care settings with which CMHCs can form and have formed linkages will differ in their organization, mandate, and the populations they serve. Each type, however, provides the CMHC with potentially greater access to citizens in need of mental health services.

Primary Health Care Centers (PHCCs)

Primary health care centers, also known as neighborhood health centers or family health centers in some areas, originated in the mid-1960s as part of a Federal Office of Economic Opportunity initiative to provide medical services to low-income urban and rural areas (Langston, 1979). These programs were expanded in the 1970s to include special initiatives focusing on the delivery of primary health care services to rural, migrant, and poor urban areas that were medically underserved (Ozarin, Samuels, & Biedenkapp, 1978). Presently, there are approximately 1000 federally sponsored PHCCs in the country, many of which are organized to provide services in multiple satellite sites.

PHCCs are intended to offer a comprehensive range of primary health and health-related social services, including preventive health care, 24-hour diagnosis and treatment of uncomplicated illnesses, outreach and home health services, dental care, and mental health services. Not all of these services have to be provided in one setting. Rather, PHCCs are to make maximum use of existing services in their area to ensure *comprehensive primary care* while using linkages to ensure patient access to more specialized and intensive secondary and tertiary care, including extended diagnosis, long-term care, and inpatient treatment.

Health Maintenance Organizations (HMOs)

HMOs are prepaid health care delivery systems in which the subscriber is eligible to receive a predetermined range and amount of services. A federally qualified HMO must provide subscribers unlimited visits to the primary care physicians and up to 20 visits to mental health clinicians (Coleman, 1980). As is the case in PHCCs, HMOs can arrange for care, including secondary and tertiary care, through referral and/or subcontracts with other providers and facilities.

General Hospitals and Emergency Rooms

The organizational structure and operation of general hospitals lend themselves to include mental health as part of the range of services available. Often, however, the emphasis is exclusively on inpatient psychiatric beds and, in some cases, minimal psychiatric-liaison consultation to other depart-

---

TABLE 9.1   Potential Benefits of Health and Mental Health Linkages

---

1. *Increased Accessibility*
   a. Improved geographical and cultural accessibility
   b. Decreased waiting times
   c. Reduced stigma associated with receiving mental health services
   d. Reduced mystery surrounding the process of mental health care

2. *Improved Case-Finding, Utilization, and Continuity*
   a. Improved detection of general mental health problems by primary care providers
   b. Improved ability to detect and meet specialized needs of high-risk groups (e.g., elderly, poor, bereaved)
   c. Increased diagnostic precision through education and consultation by mental health staff
   d. Improved medical care for psychiatric patients
   e. Improvement in the balance of medication and counseling for primary health care patients (reduction in overuse or inappropriate use of minor/major tranquilizers)
   f. Improved patient compliance with treatment regimens, less shopping
   g. More appropriate utilization of health services by emotionally disturbed patients who tend to overutilize health care services
   h. Improved follow-up and referral over time, within families, and across providers
   i. Improved patient satisfaction

3. *Improved Synthesis of Health and Mental Health Knowledge*
   a. Improved coordination among staff and their special skills and services
   b. Increase in family-oriented health and mental health care
   c. Increased opportunities for research on cause and treatment of all illnesses

---

ments. A critical need also exists for mental health services in the hospital emergency room (see Chapter 15 in this volume).

Benefits of Health-Mental Health Linkage

Linkages between CMHCs and organized health care settings promise several kinds of benefits, summarized in Table 9.1.

Many factors limit access to mental health services. The poor match between the location of services and the location of populations most in need is particularly troublesome. Children and elderly are unable to travel distances to get care (Borus, Burns, Jacobson, Macht, Morrill, & Wilson, 1979). The problem is more acute in rural areas due to a shortage of trained personnel, great distances, and lack of transportation (Daniels, 1976; Martinez, 1979). Poverty in both rural (Flax, Wagenfeld, Ivens, & Weiss, 1979) and urban areas (Martinez, 1979) has also been cited as a barrier. Finally, and perhaps most importantly, patients perceive a stigma in being associated with mental illness and the use of services in mental health settings (Borus et al., 1979). This perception is present in the general population and is especially prevalent among some of the most high-risk groups, such as the poor, the elderly, and minorities.

Using available NIMH statistics from general hospitals, nursing homes, specialty mental health settings, and outpatient medical settings, Regier, Goldberg, and Taube (1978) estimate the national prevalence rate of mental disorders to be 15%. Of those with psychiatric disorders, 54.1% (9% of the total population) are seen *exclusively* in the primary care/outpatient medical sector and 3.4% are seen in the general hospital inpatient/nursing home care sector. Only about 15% (3% of the total population) receive care in the specialty mental health sector. Six percent receive care in both sectors. A large percentage (21.5%) cannot be accounted for and may not be in treatment or are receiving services in other types of human services agencies.

As these estimates indicate, most mentally disordered persons are already being seen in the health care sector, which therefore offers particular advantages for overcoming accessibility barriers. The decentralized and risk-targeted locations of PHCCs address geographical and cultural barriers (Borus, 1976; Morrill, 1975; Ozarin et al., 1978). Most importantly, in contrast to mental health, all types of health care settings are more attitudinally or psychologically acceptable to their intended target populations. A large-scale evaluation showed that about two-thirds of the population in their service areas use their services (Langston, 1979). This same evaluation, however, also revealed that only about one-half of PHCCs could offer mental health services. Lack of mental health services was identified as the greatest deficiency in the way PHCCs were delivering their mandated services.

The provision of mental health services within an organized health care setting will widen the portals of entry to mental health care. Brissenden and Lennard (1970) found a higher than expected rate of utilization of mental health services by traditionally underrepresented minorities when services were provided within a medical setting. In one of the few research studies in this area, Lowe (1980) found a significantly greater correlation between "need," based on demographic factors, and utilization of mental health care in colocated health/mental health settings, compared to the need-utilization correlations in free-standing mental health programs. By using a correlational time-series design to study the colocation process, he showed this improved utilization to be a function of the colocation process.

In a survey of health-mental health linkages demonstrations funded by the federal government, respondents reported an increase in primary medical care staff awareness of mental health problems (Broskowski, 1980a). Some case studies have also reported improved case-finding and early identification of emotional problems (Borus et al., 1979, Burns, 1980). Case-finding is also facilitated by outreach efforts that are needed in rural areas and in reaching the elderly (Kagarise, 1979). Improved case-finding increases the potential for preventive efforts (Morrill, 1975).

The quality of care may also be improved. Difficult-to-manage patients, like psychosomatic cases, are more effectively treated when there is coordination between health and mental health care (Pincus, 1980; for a more complete review of the patient management issues, see Hankin and Oktay's [1979] review of the literature).

Overall, there is improved utilization and efficiency in the linked care systems. There is less duplication of services (Morrill, 1978), and the services that are available are more appropriately used. Patients with emotional problems are high utilizers of medical care (Hankin & Oktay, 1979), and research has shown that the availability of mental health care in some health settings can significantly reduce medical care utilization (Jones & Vischi, 1979). The possibility that mental health services can reduce inappropriate health care costs (i.e., the cost-offset phenomenon) is explored in greater depth in Chapter 14 of this volume.

Numerous studies have examined the physician's referral practices for patients with mental disorders. Fink and Shapiro (1966) found in a group health plan that 53% of patients with mental disorders were treated with drugs alone and that another 18% were treated with drugs and referred to psychiatrists. Similarly, Locke, Krantz, and Kramer (1966) found that physicians in a prepaid group practice referred only 17% of patients with psychiatric problems. Reasons for not referring are numerous, including the belief that a psychiatric referral is unacceptable to patients and that psychiatric care is expensive and therefore not financially feasible for many patients. In addition to the expense of treatment, Gerdine and Bragg (1970) cite long waiting lists as a reason for not referring. Martinez (1979) found that community health center physicians do not refer because of a lack of communication between centers, difficulties in scheduling appointments, and lack of bilingual staff. Physician attitudes are also important in this regard. Goldberg et al. (1979) found that pediatricians believed they could handle the child's emotional problems themselves, were reluctant to label the case as mental illness, and did not want to share the responsibility for care.

Increased continuity, facilitated by linkages, can improve the coordination and referral processes. There is a lower rate of loss of patients upon referral (Borus, 1976), referrals are more frequently used, and the communication process is generally faster and more efficient.

Linkage Mechanisms and Models

Organizations can link together at a number of levels, including both administrative and direct service levels. While administrative support is necessary for a successful service linkage, interorganizational efforts at the direct service level appear to hold the greatest promise for increasing accessibility and comprehensiveness of services (John, 1977).

In their study of federally funded service integration projects, Gans and Horton (1975) developed a taxonomy of adminstrative and direct service linkage mechanisms. Based on numerous case studies, these investigators classified each linkage mechanism according to the resources and time needed for their development and their potential impact on access, continuity, and efficiency of services. For the most part, administrative linkages require longer periods of time to implement. Administrative linkages include such activities as joint budgeting, planning, funding, and consolidated personnel administration. The high cost of these forms of linkage may negate the benefits achieved (John, 1977). However, several forms of administrative linkage are more readily instituted and are hypothesized to have a high impact on services (Gans & Horton, 1975). These mechanisms are joint purchase of services, colocation of staff from autonomous agencies, and staff outstanding in the linked agency.

In general, direct service linkages require shorter implementation periods (Gans & Horton, 1975). Core service linkages involve joint outreach, intake, diagnosis, referral, and follow-up. Ongoing case coordination linkage mechanisms involve case conferences, multidisciplinary treatment teams, and the use of case managers to coordinate the provision of services by multiple autonomous service providers. Both types of direct service linkages can increase access and comprehensiveness of services, but little is known about their impact on the outcome or effectiveness of service delivery (John, 1977).

Those linkage mechanisms which appear to be most readily implemented with the greatest impact on access are the case coordination mechanisms and the core services that together form a system of case management. The administrative mechanisms that hold the most promise in this regard are those which most directly get the client in treatment and avoid higher-level agency administrative integration. They do not, however, obviate the need for administrative support if the linkage is to be successful.

This taxonomy of linkage mechanisms provides a basic but incomplete method to conceptualize linkages between CMHCs and organized health care settings. Each mechanism can be viewed as one mode for interorganizational coordination. However, these mechanisms do not occur as isolated dimensions. Rather, several types may need to exist simultaneously, forming a "system" of linked care. Such systems can themselves be classified into larger models of coordinated health and mental health care.

Levels of Care

Before presenting specific models of linkages between health and mental health settings, it will be useful to consider a broader context of coordinated health and mental health care suggested by Macht (1975). Macht conceptualized four levels of mental health care, each to be provided in different types of settings.

Level I care, or primary mental health services, would be delivered at the neighborhood level, within organized health or multiservice centers serving 10,000 to 50,000 persons. Services at this level would include direct clinical care on an outpatient basis, consultation and education, preventive efforts, crisis intervention, and aftercare programs. Level II care, or acute secondary mental health services, would take place in community hospitals or CMHCs, covering a service area population of up to 200,000 persons. These services would include short-term hospitalization and areawide direct and consultation services. Level III care, or extended secondary mental health services, would take place in the same settings as Level II services. Level III services would include specialized inpatient care of less than 12 months and more specialized outpatient services. Finally, Level IV care, or tertiary mental health services, would be provided for persons needing long-term inpatient care or custodial care at regional facilities serving two service areas at a minimum.

The success of this system of care would rely heavily on linkages between service providers both within and across levels of care. At this point we will focus on those linkage mechanisms that operate at the level of primary mental health services (Level I). Several models have been proposed, ranging from simple interorganizational referral agreements to extensively integrated, single-setting service systems.

Linkage Models

Pincus (1980) proposed a highly generalizable linkage model, applicable to a broad range of settings and to systems of coordinated care that can, but do not necessarily, involve separate organizations. Pincus conceptualizes three critical dimensions which can operate in different combinations to produce at least six distinctive models. Each dimension may be formally or informally specified in the linkage arrangement. The first dimension consists of the "contractual elements" of the linkage agreement. These specify the content of the linkage both in terms of what linkage mechanisms will be included in the agreement and how they will operate. Thus, this dimension includes the mechanisms of patient referral and follow-up as well as such administrative mechanisms as record sharing, billing and financial procedures, and joint planning and program supervision.

The second dimension consists of the "functional elements" of the linkage. These are the actual services, and the staff who provide them, that grow out of the linkage arrangement and are directly encountered by the patients.

The third dimension consists of the "educational elements." These include all aspects of the linkage arrangement that enhance the health care provider's knowledge and skill in mental health, as well as the mental health provider's understanding of health care.

The first of six models described by Pincus (1980) is called the Agreement Model, in which the primary and almost exclusive focus is on the contractual elements of the linkage. Mechanisms of patient referral and follow-up are specified between at least two organizations, but there are no joint services provided, so no functional elements are involved. Educational elements, if they occur, are the result of informal feedback during the referral process. Examples of this model include the relationship between CMHCs and private medical practitioners, and between CMHCs and HMOs where the HMO contracts to purchase services on a referral basis. In these examples, the patient has the major responsibility for utilizing the referral and connecting the two systems.

The Triage Model has more articulated contractual elements and adds a functional component. In this case, a staff person is designated who performs the liaison functions of triage, referral, and follow-up between the agencies. The presence of a mental health professional in the health care agency may involve educational elements, but these are secondary. An example of this model is the CMHC-PHCC linkage initiative recently developed by the federal government. (See Chapter 2 of this volume.) These linkages involve a formal, written agreement between the agencies and the presence of a mental health professional who performs the liaison functions noted above.

The third model is called the Service Delivery Team. This model is characterized predominantly by a range of direct services provided by a mental health unit under the auspices of a health care organization. The contractual elements are well articulated, since both health and mental health systems are under the auspices of a single organization. The educational elements are similar to those of the Triage Model, but may be more extensive due to the greater number of mental health personnel within the health care setting. Examples of this model are group health plans, HMOs, and PHCCs with their own mental health units whose primary purpose is the delivery of direct service to patients. (See Chapter 6 by Budman for more information on HMOs.)

The Consultation and Service Model has a greater emphasis on educational elements while maintaining an emphasis on functional elements as well. As in the previous model, there is a specific unit that provides specialty mental health services. In this model, however, greater emphasis is placed on case consultation so that the mental health capabilities of the primary care provider are enhanced. When needed, the mental health personnel provide specialty services directly to the patient. Examples of this model are teaching hospitals with consultation-liaison programs and some HMOs.

The fifth model is called the Supervision and Education Model. As the name implies, this model's primary emphasis is on educational elements. The goal is to furnish primary care providers with the ability to assess and treat patients with emotional problems, as well as the ability to know when a specialty referral is needed. There may be some minimal contractual elements, while the functional elements are the services and referrals provided by the primary care staff. Examples of this model are continuing education for nonpsychiatric medical staff and special programs in graduate medical education.

The final model, the Integrated Health Care Team, is a synthesis of all three types of elements. Rather than forming a separate entity, the mental health staff are thoroughly integrated into the primary health care teams. Through regular team meetings, referrals, case consultations, and specialty backup services are made available to the patient. The relationship of members of the team is well specified, yet allows for flexibility in case management. Examples of this model can be found in HMOs and in some PHCCs.

The models developed by Pincus are the most general and widely applicable to settings where health and mental health linkages are desired. In addition, these models are more comprehensive than those presented by others, as they incorporate administrative factors, clinical or service factors, and staffing and training considerations. Unfortunately, the level of generality of these models makes them less useful for detailed planning of a specific linkage between a CMHC and some other health setting.

A set of models more specific to CMHC and PHCC linkages was developed by Borus and his colleagues (1975). These investigators surveyed 19 neighborhood health centers (NHC) in the Boston area that had some type of mental health services. Based on the nature of their organizational relationships, and the relative contribution of resources by the CMHC and the NHC, they identified four models that described these programs.

The most prevalent model was called Joint Endeavor. In these settings the NHC houses a neighborhood *mental* health program and directly employs some of the mental health staff, mainly indigenous professionals and paraprofessionals. Additional professional-level staff are employed by the CMHC and are delegated to work within the NHC. These Joint Endeavor programs have varying degrees of autonomy and back-up linkages to the CMHC.

The Autonomous NHC model is characterized by a mental health program that is funded and run totally by the NHC. These programs may be either part-time or full-time depending on the level of funds available to the NHC for such services. Nonmonetary liaison to the local CMHC, presumably for referral to more specialized care, is also a characteristic of these settings.

When the entire staff of the mental health program located within the NHC are employees of the CMHC, the model is called a Community Mental Health Outpost. Finally, the Consultative Model is characterized by the lack of any mental health program in the NHC; the NHC has a "working alliance" with a nearby CMHC satellite that serves the same area. The relationship is solely for purposes of consultation and referral to the CMHC.

While the models presented by Borus et al. are more specific to NHC and CMHC linkages, they do not clearly describe the specific mechanisms of the interaction between the centers involved. Health care teams, case managers, and a joint health-mental health record may be maintained, but these mechanisms are not related to any particular model. The main determinant of each model appears to be who hires or contributes mental health staff to the program. Contribution of space, funds, and other resources receives little emphasis. As occurs in Pincus's models, decision rules for classifying a program into one of the models are absent, making the Borus et al. models difficult to use for future planning and research purposes.

A "family health care team" model has been suggested by Morrill (1972) as the most appropriate for mental health care in an NHC. Similarly, Coleman and Patrick (1976) have recommended a "team collaboration model" for use in HMOs. Other models briefly discussed by these authors are the use of psychiatric consultants, educating primary care clinicians, and a full-time program similar to the Autonomous Model of Borus et al. (1975). All of these models are dismissed by Coleman and Patrick (1976) as being ineffective in the long run and a continuation of fragmented, separated systems of care.

There is a difference between the team models proposed by Morrill (1972) and that of Coleman and Patrick (1976). Morrill recommends an integrated team in which the mental health professional provides diagnostic and therapeutic services within the team as well as referring patients to more centralized specialty services. The mental health professional takes an egalitarian role in the team. In contrast, the team model recommended by Coleman and Patrick (1976) places the primary care physician in a central role, since he or she is the most visible and accessible member of the health care team (Coleman, 1979). Only patients needing specialized care are referred to the mental health team member. Economic considerations make this team configuration more suitable to an HMO, since enrollees are entitled to unlimited visits to physicians with only more limited visits to mental health specialists.

Burns (1980) presented a case study of a successful health/mental health linkage within a neighborhood health center. She itemized eleven specific mechanisms for coordination and examples of each, summarized in Table 9.2.

Selection of Models and Mechanisms

The models and mechanisms reviewed range from extensively integrated, single-setting programs based on well-coordinated, joint endeavors

TABLE 9.2   Approaches for Health/Mental Health Interaction
at the Provider Level

Vehicles for Health/Mental Health Coordination	Examples of Applications
1. Single medical record	Formal communication among providers
2. Multi-discipline health care team	Multiproblem families with health and mental health problems are frequently presented
3. Ease of referral to mental health services	Open intake system by mental health service
4. Case-centered consultation	Health provider requests advice on management of patients
5. Center committees	Medical records, various task forces
6. Inservice education	Series on alcoholism, child development, infant-parent relationships
7. Joint patient interview	Modeling assessment approaches for health providers
8. Collaborative program	Preschool screening, obesity group, medication clinic
9. Client-centered consultation	Pediatric nurses counseling adolescent mothers meet with psychiatrist regularly
10. Liaison to units	A pediatrician attends the child mental health intake meeting
11. Collaborative research	A study of internists' patterns for prescribing tranquilizers

between two organizations, to loosely integrated linkages between separate agencies involving infrequent and informal referral and consultation. When two or more agencies are involved, the degree of symmetry, or relative contribution and control of resources by each organization, becomes another important dimension of linkage selection (Broskowski, 1980a). It is unfortunate, however, that there is little in the literature to suggest which dimensions or models are best for different settings or goals.

Pincus (1980) lists six factors that must be considered when developing a linkage program, but does not specify how they affect model selection. These factors are: (1) characteristics and needs of the people served; (2) geographical and cultural constraints; (3) the location and auspices of functional elements; (4) available financing mechanisms; (5) staff attitudes and philosophy of care; and (6) level of care provided by the linkage. The only specific suggestion Pincus offers is that models emphasizing educational elements will not work in fee-for-service settings, since consultation, supervision, and education are not reimbursable activities.

Coleman and Patrick (1976) recommend a particular team configuration in an HMO. Morrill (1975) argues for the use of teams in general, especially in large settings where separate health and mental health units would result in poor communication and coordination of care. These colocated teams, however, will have a much greater chance of success when considered in the early planning stages of new facilities (Broskowski, 1980b). Colocation of services might be the organization of choice in rural areas where distances between centers make referral more difficult. The models described by Borus et al. (1975) are probably most appropriate for urban areas, in which they were observed, due to the greater availability of resources which they require. Within any model, the choice of mechanisms, such as those described by Burns (1980), will depend upon administrative and clinical interests.

At this point, we should not assume that all potential models have been described. The ones presently available in the literature do not adequately describe *both administrative and clinical concerns*, the relation between these, or the potential time and costs involved. When agencies are planning a linkage, it would probably be best to start with some of the less expensive mechanisms for linkage, such as the direct service mechanisms discussed earlier. This approach would allow for an assessment of the potential advantages of more expensive linkages before committing a great deal of resources.

At this point, it would be useful to consider the general and specific issues involved in linkage development and maintenance in order to provide a framework in which to plan, implement, manage, and evaluate linkage projects.

Issues in Developing and Maintaining Linkages

Despite the legal mandates, incentives, and potential advantages for integrated health and mental health delivery, there remain serious barriers to the development of effective linkages. Some of the issues which must be considered include those general factors that can inhibit or facilitate any type of interorganizational relationship, as well as concerns specific to the nature of health and mental health coordination.

In a recent review of the literature on interorganizational relationships, Broskowski (1980b) identified a list of five environmental, six intraorganizational, and twenty interorganizational factors that can inhibit or facilitate linkages between organizations. These 31 factors must be considered by any set of organizations considering the development of linkages. Although they are listed separately here in summary form, most of these variables are interdependent and interact with one another in complex and poorly understood ways.

Environmental Factors

The major environmental factors affecting linkages are the amount and location of available resources and the rate of environmental change, complexity, and predictability. An environment characterized by scarce resources, clustered or organized in a few locations, with intermediate levels of complexity, predictability, and change facilitates the development of linkages. Abundant resources in a highly predictable, simple, and stable environment inhibit the development of linkages, since each organization can afford autonomous activities.

Intraorganizational Factors

While infrequently considered, characteristics *within* an organization will affect its general ability and willingness to develop and maintain linkages. An organization that is well organized and coordinated internally and that has an advanced capacity to collect, process, store, retrieve, and distribute information internally will be more capable of developing external linkages with minimal internal disruption and conflict.

The nature of an organization's primary service technology will also affect its relationships with other agencies. Services based on sequential processing of standardized units (e.g., food stamp services) lend themselves to linkages at the front and back ends more readily than do intensive service technologies; those based on unpredictable scheduling and sequencing of multiple personnel and other resources (e.g., emergency room services) to serve nonstandardized cases. The latter types of technologies suggest greater needs for internal control of all the needed resources than one can generally achieve through a linkage.

Internal leadership styles are also critical. Managing a complex organization based on a strategy of multiple relationships for critical resources requires a leadership style that is highly flexible, innovative, and tolerant toward change. Finally, when an organization has abundant resources of its own, over which it has unfettered control, it is less inclined to develop linkages. On the other hand, if it has only limited control over very scarce resources, it will also avoid the risks of a linkage where it is likely to be dominated. Linkages are facilitated when there are intermediate levels of resources and control.

Interorganizational Factors

The last set of conditions affecting linkages are interorganizational factors. These can be subdivided into those that *compare* the potential linking organizations on various dimensions and those that look at the existing or potential *relationships* between the organizations. The comparative conditions will be summarized first.

Dissimilarities between the organizations in terms of size, structure, and technology add to the complexity of any relationship, as does the sheer number of organizations involved. As the complexity increases, the probability of a successful linkage being formed decreases. However, if the organizations involved are mutually interdependent, have complementary and not competitive service goals, and similar philosophies of service, then a linkage will be facilitated. Furthermore, support from common higher-level fundings, regulatory, or sanctioning agencies, that still allows for voluntary involvement, will increase the probability of a successful linkage being formed. Linkages are also more likely if the agencies involved have had positive prior linkage experiences with other agencies.

The conditions that characterize the relationship between organizations, or relational factors, are also affected by prior linkage experience. In this case, positive prior interaction with a particular organization will increase the likelihood of continuing or forming additional linkages with that organization. When linkages are reciprocally planned and negotiated, and formalized to the point of allowing written specification and standardization of what is to be exchanged, the linkage will have a better chance of being successful. If the exchange yields equal benefits for both agencies and is conducted over small distances on a relatively frequent basis, linkage will also be facilitated. Finally, gradual but firm implementation of the linkage and a formal commitment of resources to manage it will aid in its development. Effective linkages are also characterized by continuing and mutual exchange of information between the organizations. This feedback is used to refine or reformulate their linkages plans as problems arise. It is critical that linkage planning and implementation receives support from top levels of both organizations.

There is little in the published literature to suggest how a linkage should be planned or implemented, but it is clear that a number of factors will facilitate the process. Well-defined goals and written agreements that make explicit the areas of responsibility, authority, and benefits for each organization are helpful. A phased implementation, starting with the least costly modes of coordination, will help in securing further commitment to the linkage process.

As can be seen from this brief summary of general factors affecting linkages, the process of developing, implementing, and managing linkages is complex and requires consideration of numerous factors. The process can be especially difficult in developing linkages between PHCCs and CMHCs, since these organizations start at a disadvantage with respect to a number of the general factors summarized above.

Specific CMHC-PHCC Linkage Concerns

The case report and research literatures on health and mental health linkages (Broskowski, 1980a, 1980b) reflect the full spectrum of possible linkage mechanisms, ranging from simple information and referral agreements to intermittent liaison arrangements, full-time linkage workers, separate mental health teams, and integrated health and mental health teams. The specific factors influencing these linkages can be summarized according to environmental conditions and administrative and clinical concerns.

Earls (1979) presents a vivid case study of a linkage effort that failed. One among many reasons was the instability of the local community. Racial tensions, population migration, discontinuity in neighborhood leadership, and lack of federal, state, and local government regulatory consensus combined to undermine the project. Community instability also stimulated intra-organizational turbulence, administrative confusion, and staff dissension.

Community instability does not necessarily lead to failure if a community crisis is used as an opportunity for creating change. Leadership, consensus, and consistency, however, appear critical. Poor cooperation among levels of government or between government agencies within any given level will make linkage difficult, if not impossible. The case report literature and research reveals no consistent pattern of such environmental dimensions as rural-urban, rich-poor, or resourceful-disadvantaged being related to health-mental health linkage development.

Administrative issues, internal to each agency or across the two agencies, can be critical. Administrative procedures need to be mutually well planned and explicit. Many case studies advise *written* agreements on such issues as who pays for what types of cost items (e.g., space, travel, personnel); who collects and retains which fees; whose personnel policies guide staff behavior, salary levels, and fringe benefits; and who is responsible for collecting, storing, and reporting information or other reports. While these issues may be developed over time and in an incremental fashion, based on experience and shared feedback, they should be reduced to writing.

Administrative leadership and support is consistently reported as essential. Clinical linkage staff must be sensitive to the administrators' concerns and expect, in return, adequate support to solve major or minor logistical problems. Like the external environment of both agencies, it helps if the internal environments of each are stable and well organized.

Fiscal concerns emerge because of very different philosophies and procedures with respect to billing and collecting for health and mental health services. Some linkage worker activities may not be billable (such as case consultation and training), and this can aggravate administrative concerns for cost or productivity (Schniewind, 1976; Burns, 1980). Issues of costs and reimbursement will also vary by type of setting, such as a public health clinic or a health maintenance organization.

A major administrative concern is the delineation of authority and agency autonomy. Fear of lost autonomy can be a common barrier to entering into a linkage, although Broskowski (1980a) found little reported concern for autonomy among health and mental health center directors receiving linkage demonstration funds. Some directors, however, did report problems in working out agreements for joint program planning, decision-making, and the linkage worker's job responsibilities.

Clinical concerns are more commonly reported in the case study literature (Broskowski, 1980b). The type and range of services provided through a linkage and the training, skills, and experience of linkage staff are frequent concerns. Two of the best case studies that illustrate such issues are provided by Schniewind (1976) and Burns (1980).

Productivity and direct services to clients are important legitimizing processes that mental health linkage workers must consider. Linkage staff may be tested by health staff who have unrealistically high expectations or excessively negative attitudes toward mental health professionals. Care must be taken to avoid physician resentment of mental health professionals who work on a case consultation basis. Such professionals run the risk of being seen as removed from the realities of the clinical care process and unwilling to "get their hands dirty" in direct service. The linkage staffs' clinical authority, vis-à-vis patients or other staff, must be made clear. Authority, responsibility, and supervision are generally evolutionary and developmental processes, and formal orientations and role negotiations must be carried out continuously.

Disciplinary tensions and hierarchical traditions can vary considerably across two agencies, and the linkage staff must be tolerant, patient, and flexible. Some tolerance for ambiguity is preferable. Supervisory tensions can easily emerge if linkage staff have multiple clinical and/or administrative supervisors across two or more settings. Dual-agency allegiances and staff cooptation are problematic.

Linkage staff must also work hard to maintain their own disciplinary identity and career development. Being the only mental health staff in a health setting can stimulate a sense of isolation and self-doubt. Maintaining ties to colleagues and continuing career education are two types of possible support.

Technological and ideological differences can also produce problems. Health settings typically differ from mental health settings in the volume, scheduling, and length of patient visits or total episodes of care, and in the relationship of the patient to the staff. Health settings have many visits, brief visits (10-15 minutes), and intermittent visits spread throughout the year. Many, if not most, visits are not scheduled. Privacy may be lacking, and interruptions are common. Mental health staff who are used to, or insist on, scheduled, uninterrupted, 50-minute sessions with patients are in for a surprise and possible resentment. Brief and frequent hallway meetings, non-jargon medical records notes, and on-the-spot case consultations are routine. Technologies of drugs and surgery may conflict with "talking" therapies.

Finally, true integration of health and mental health staff and services will depend on sufficient opportunities to communicate and share feedback. Colocation in shared or adjacent offices is one helpful step for this to occur. Joint inservice training, a single record system, standard referral forms, integrated committees and special project teams, and collaborative research efforts will strengthen the linkage (Burns, 1980).

Conclusions and Implications for Coordinated Care

Given the categorical nature of the human service delivery system, forming linkages between CMHCs and organized health care settings for the delivery of primary mental health services can allow these agencies to maintain their individual identities while improving the access, efficiency, and comprehensiveness of care. The potential benefits are likely to be greatest as the linkage mechanism moves from simple referral agreements toward colocated and integrated health-mental health staff teams.

Clinical and economic factors are likely to point in the direction of increasingly integrated primary health and mental health care services, with strong referral linkages for access to more intensive and specialized mental health services, similar to the integrated network of health and mental health services proposed by Macht (1975). Integrated settings, however, require a major investment of resources by both organizations, as well as administrative skill and leadership. Funds, technical assistance, and special staff training will be needed to realize a well-integrated system. While plagued by interorganizational and clinical difficulties, linkages are a feasible first step in experimenting with new forms of improved coordinated care.

References

Borus, J. Neighborhood health centers as providers of primary mental health care. *New England Journal of Medicine,* 1976, 295,140-145.

Borus, J., Burns, B., Jacobson, A., Macht, L., Morrill, R., & Wilson, E. Coordinated mental health care in neighborhood health centers. In *Mental health services in general health care, vol. 2.* Washington, DC: Institute of Medicine, National Academy of Sciences, 1979.

Borus, J., Janowitch, L., Kieffer, F., Morrill, R., Reich, L., Simone, E., & Towle, L. The coordination of mental health services at the neighborhood level. *American Journal of Psychiatry,* 1975, 132, 1177-1181.

Brissenden, R., & Lennard, H. Organization in mental health services and its effect on the treatment career of the patient. *Mental Hygiene,* 1970, 54, 416-420.

Broskowski, A. Evaluation of the primary health care project-community mental health center linkage initiative: Final report. Rockville, MD: National Institute of Mental Health, 1980.(a)

Broskowski, A. Literature review on interorganizational relationships and their relevance to health and mental health coordination. Final contract report, Contract No. 278-79-0030(OP). Rockville, MD: National Institute of Mental Health, 1980. (b)

Burns, B. A neighborhood health center model of integrated and linked health and mental health services. In *Mental health services in primary care settings: Report of a conference.* DHHS Publication No. (ADM) 80-995. Washington, DC: Government Printing Office, 1980.

Coleman, J. Treatment of emotional problems by primary physicians in an HMO. In *Mental health services in primary care settings: Report of a conference.* DHHS Publication No. (ADM) 80-995. Washington, DC: Government Printing Office, 1980.

Coleman, J., & Patrick, D. Integrating mental health services into primary medical care. *Medical Care,* 1976, 14, 654-661.

Daniels, D. The community mental health center in the rural area: Is the present model appropriate? *American Journal of Psychiatry,* 1976, 124, 32-37.

Earls, F. Experience in primary mental health care. *Journal of the National Medical Association,* 1979, 71, 779-782.

Fink, R., & Shapiro, S. Patterns of medical care related to mental illness. *Journal of Health and Human Behavior,* 1966, 7, 98-105.

Flax, J., Wagenfeld, M., Ivens, R., & Weiss, R. *Mental health and rural America: An overview and annotated bibliography.* Washington, DC: National Institute of Mental Health, 1979.

Gans, S., & Horton, G. *Integration of human services.* New York: Praeger, 1975.

Gerdine, M., & Bragg, R. Referral patterns among mental health agents in three suburban communities. *American Journal of Orthopsychiatry,* 1970, 40, 841-849.

Goldberg, I., Regier, D., McInerny, T., Pless, I., & Roghmann, K. The role of the pediatrician in the delivery of mental health services to children. *Pediatrics,* 1979, 63, 898-909.

Hankin, J., & Oktay, J. *Mental disorder and primary medical care: An analytical review of the literature.* NIMH Monograph Series D, No. 5. DHEW Publication No. (ADM) 78-661. Washington, DC: Government Printing Office, 1979.

John, D. *Managing the human service system: What have we learned from services integration?* Human Services Monograph Series, No. 4, Project SHARE. Rockville, MD: National Institute of Mental Health, 1977.

Jones, K., & Vischi, T. Impact of alcohol, drug abuse, and mental health treatment on medical care utilization: A review of the research literature. *Medical Care,* 1979, 17 (Supplement).

Kagarise, M. The interface between primary mental health care and primary medical services: A fruitful area for the establishment of interorganizational linkages. North Carolina Division of Mental Health and Mental Retardation and Substance Abuse Services, 1979.

Langston, J. The neighborhood health center program. In J. Abert (Ed.), *Program evaluation at HEW.* New York: Marcel Dekker, 1979.

Locke, B., Krantz, G., & Kramer, M. Psychiatric need and demand in a prepaid group practice program. *American Journal of Public Health,* 1966, 56, 895-904.

Lowe, B. An evaluation of the impact of providing mental health services in neighborhood health centers on utilization by community residents in need of service. Ph.D. dissertation, Miami University, Oxford, Ohio, 1980.

Macht, L. Beyond the mental health center: Planning for a community of neighborhoods. *Psychiatric Annals,* 1975, 5, 56-69.

Martinez, L. Factors relating to the delivery of mental health services in community health centers. Unpublished manuscript, Office of Planning, Evaluation, and Legislation, Health Services Administration, Washington, D.C., 1979.

Morrill, R. A new mental health services model for the comprehensive neighborhood health center. *American Journal of Public Health,* 1972, 62, 1108-1111.

Morrill, R. Comprehensive mental health through a neighborhood health center. In E. Lieberman (Ed.), *Mental health: The public health challenge.* Washington, DC: American Public Health Association, 1975.

Morrill, R. The future for mental health in primary health care programs. *American Journal of Psychiatry,* 1978, 135, 1351-1355.

Ozarin, L., Samuels, M., & Biedenkapp, J. Need for mental health services in federally funded rural primary health care systems. *Public Health Reports,* 1978, 93, 351-355.

Pincus, H. Linking general health and mental health systems of care: Conceptual models of implementation. *American Journal of Psychiatry,* 1980, 137, 315-320.

President's Commission on Mental Health. Report to the President, vol. 1. Washington, DC: Government Printing Office, 1978.

Regier, D., Goldberg, I., & Taube, C. The de facto U.S. mental health system: A public health perspective. *Archives of General Psychiatry,* 1978, 35, 685-693.

Schniewind, H. A psychiatrist's experience in a primary health care setting. *International Journal of Psychiatry in Medicine,* 1976, 7, 229-240.

III

TRAINING FOR COORDINATED CARE

10

Integrating Health-Mental Health Training

Linda Heard Hollen
Robert P. Ehrlich
Northside Community Mental Health Center,
Tampa, Florida

Stephen L. White
Pawtucket-Central Falls Community
Mental Health Center,
Pawtucket, Rhode Island

The U.S. health manpower strategy from the 1940s through the 1960s focused on increasing the supply of health care professionals in a variety of specialty areas (Adams & Cheney, 1979; Regier & Rosenfeld, 1977). The prevailing hope was that increased numbers of specialty service providers would attenuate problems in both health and mental health care delivery systems. As a result, the thrust of training initiatives was in the direction of producing health care providers with distinct constellations of skills. The 1970s, however, heralded the need for a new direction in manpower training and development in all areas of health care provision and, more specifically, in terms of mental health and health care linkages. The genesis of this new direction was influenced by a number of significant events.

First, larger numbers of mental health professionals did not, as expected, satisfy the demands of individuals with mental health needs in all geographical areas. In addition, despite the availability of mental health specialists, studies indicated that individuals overwhelmingly continued to be treated by their primary care physician when an emotional difficulty became evident (Hankin & Oktay, 1979; Regier, Goldberg, & Taube, 1978). In particular, among the roughly 15 percent of Americans who are diagnosed as having a mental disorder, about four times as many are treated by primary care physicians as by mental health specialists (Brown & Regier, 1977).

Similarly, in a recent review article White (1981) discussed data indicating that individuals experiencing mental health problems utilize significantly higher levels of expensive medical diagnostic and treatment services, and that the utilization rate tends to decrease when mental health services are made available. Chapter 4 of this volume reviews such findings in greater detail. Nevertheless, these data lend credence to the notion that health and mental health are indeed indivisible. Both are essential and interacting aspects of the total person. Accordingly, the nation's health manpower strategy has begun to shift from developing larger numbers of more specialized professionals to emphasizing a more integrated approach.

As early as 1973, the World Health Organization predicted that the primary care physician would play a major role in mental health care to the point of becoming the "Keystone of Community Psychiatry" (WHO, 1973). In 1976, the National Institute of Mental Health called for the establishment of the Workgroup on Mental Health Training of Primary Care Providers (Regier & Rosenfeld, 1977). Furthermore, the American Psychological Association has established a Health Psychology Division, while the National Association of Social Work has organized a Health-Mental Health Task Force. Moreover, the Institute of Medicine conducted a conference in April 1979 dealing with mental health services in primary care settings (Institute of Medicine, 1979).

Indicators in both the private and public sector demonstrate that this integrationist approach is taking hold. For example, the Health Professions Educational Assistance Act of 1978 (PL 94-484) supports an increase in the relative proportion of primary care physicians compared with specialists. In addition, the Mental Health Systems Act of 1980 (PL 96-398) provides for grants to assist health care centers in providing mental health services to their patients. Likewise, family practice residencies, now required to have a psychiatry and behavioral sciences component to their curriculum, have flourished in recent years.

Clearly, if the integrationist trend continues to supplant previous health manpower strategies, the training curriculum of all germane disciplines must respond to this once implicit call. The disciplines which need to be most intimately involved in bringing this goal to fruition are social work, psychology, psychiatry, and primary care medicine. Accordingly, this chapter will discuss issues pertaining to the role of each of these disciplines in providing the necessary training. In addition, two model training programs seeking to foster a more integrated health care approach will be described, and recommendations will be offered regarding future research and training efforts.

Social Work

We can trace the involvement of social workers in primary health care settings back to 1918, a watershed year for the emerging profession. Thousands of casualties were returning from the war that raged in Europe; there were epidemics of tuberculosis, polio, and venereal disease; and even more devastating, there was a pandemic of influenza (Kerson, 1979). In addition, leaders of the social work community were among the first to embrace psychoanalytic thought in the United States. These factors led to the establishment of schools of social work at Smith College and Simmons College, both of which had close ties with Boston hospitals. The early focus of the profession was on the psychosocial needs of patients and their families whose work and routine lives had been disrupted by war wounds and illnesses for which there were inadequate treatments. Attempts were made to reduce stress and anxiety by using psychoanalytic techniques to help people adjust to their wounds, illnesses, and reduced economic circumstances.

Shortly after World War I, the social work profession virtually split into two tracks: medical and psychiatric. Medical social workers worked in hospitals, while psychiatric social workers worked in the newly emerging child guidance centers in state hospitals. While psychiatric social work was decidedly more prestigious, medical social work remained a strong component of the profession. Along with other major changes in the social work profession during the 1960s, many medical *and* psychiatric social workers, now calling themselves clinical social workers, came together. They formed new societies and founded journals to promote a greater knowledge base for social workers in health and mental health settings, and to discover innovative ways of responding to the health needs of the nation (Falck, 1978; Goldberg, 1973). While the medical social work literature is largely confined to case studies, it is clear that the profession is making important contributions to working with the psychosocial concomitants of physical illnesses (Cain, 1974; Sokol, 1976; Morse, 1974). An excellent handbook dealing with the practice of social work in community health settings has been prepared by Kumabe and associates (1977).

Two important aspects of social work intervention in health care settings are the focus on the prevention of psychological problems that could emanate from physical problems and the involvement of the patient's whole family in such interventions. These are two areas that are difficult for traditional primary health care personnel to address due to their work style and specialized training. For example, primary health care personnel commonly focus on specific medical problems in the context of a busy, often chaotic, daily schedule that rotates around very brief (10-15 minute) patient contacts.

Clinical social workers are becoming increasingly important members of health care teams in hospitals (Nieman & Hoops, 1977; Sokol, 1976) and in private medical practices (Korpela, 1973). Some of the most promising recent contributions of clinical social workers to improve health-mental health linkages have been in the area of training primary health care personnel. Hanna and Schachter (1979) describe a course taught by social workers to medical students and family practice residents in a Canadian medical school. The course covers basic aspects of human psychosocial growth and development, doctor-patient interactions, and the empathic and professional use of oneself in dealing with patients. The course is designed to sensitize doctors to the psychosocial needs of their patients and to prepare them to respond to those needs. Even more widespread, although underreported in the literature, are the contributions of clinical social workers to the clinical training of medical students and primary care residents (see, for example, Korpela, 1973).

Psychology

Psychologists are not newcomers to health care settings; their assessment, diagnostic, and consultative skills have long been relied upon by medical personnel. However, the interest in and demand for psychologists in health care settings has been growing dramatically during the past decade (Olbrisch & Sechrest, 1979). This trend is largely attributable to the widespread recognition that psychologists can contribute to the quality of health care in many more ways than had previously been assumed. In addition to continuing to perform their traditional functions, psychologists are now becoming involved in a substantially broader range of health care settings and are serving in expanded and innovative roles. For example, Chapter 12 of this volume describes their potential role as researchers of health service systems, ranging from etiology to service delivery.

A brief review of a recent special issue of *Professional Psychology* (August 1979), entirely devoted to psychologists in health care settings, provides some appreciation for the breadth of this trend. Examples are presented of psychologists functioning in health maintenance organizations (Budman and Clifford, 1979), family practices (Bibace & Walsh, 1979), nursing homes (Lebray, 1979), hospitals (Bloom, 1979), rehabilitation centers (Grzesiak, 1979), public health organizations (Stone, 1979), dentists' offices (Sachs, 1979), children's hospitals (Wright, 1979), and other community settings. Within these settings, the diversity of roles and functions served by psychologists is remarkable. These include administrator, teacher, supervisor, clinical consultant, organizational consultant, clinician, liaison, referral agent, researcher, program planner and developer, assessor, evaluator, and patient advocate. Psychologists in these settings were also involved in the treatment of health problems which include, among many others, pain, hypertension, smoking, stress, obesity, pediatric cancer, myocardial infarction, and asthma.

With the increased likelihood that psychologists will be called upon to serve supportive or primary roles in health care settings, it is necessary for graduate training programs in psychology to assess the extent to which their curricula prepare graduates for those roles. This assessment requires answering such preliminary questions as: What is health psychology? What do health psychologists do? What will health psychologists be doing in the future? How is being a health psychologist the same as or different from practicing other relevant types of psychology? In other words, operationalizing the concept of health psychology and its practice must precede the assessment of a program's current status. Following this preliminary task, the next step would be to determine the program's commitment to developing a health psychology component within the curriculum and providing the resources available to accomplish the desired level of involvement. The commitment and resources may range from merely tailoring the current curriculum to highlight its adaptability to health issues, to offering specific health psychology courses, to adding a specialized practicum or internship, to creating a separate health psychology program.

Stone (1979) described the evolution and current status of a specialized doctoral program in health psychology at the University of California, San Francisco (see Chapter 12). Located within the school of medicine, the program concentrates on research of the health care systems and emphasizes "the psychological aspects of the health care process—the cognitive, personality, and social psychological issues that effect the outcomes of health transactions" (p. 599). The three major guidelines proposed by the author for establishing a curriculum are that the graduates should first and foremost be psychologists; that they should primarily be researchers, utilizing empirically-based approaches to consult with and train health care professionals; and that they must understand the social and biomedical aspects of health care environments in order to be accepted as peers and gain respect from other health care personnel.

While a few graduate and postdoctoral health psychology programs have already been developed, most psychology departments will not have the resources necessary to establish specialized training. The majority of psychologists currently working in medical settings have been trained in traditional graduate programs. Given the limited availability of specialty programs, in combination with the projected need for health psychologists, it is probable that the pattern of limited resources will continue (Olbrisch & Sechrest, 1979). Thus, the problem confronting most graduate programs will be determining how to reallocate resources, or utilize existing resources more efficiently in order to provide subspecialty training in health psychology.

Olbrisch and Sechrest (1979) have outlined several concrete suggestions for enlisting psychology department resources, university-wide resources, and community resources. On the departmental level, students can be encouraged to design health psychology projects that are related to the faculty's existing specialized areas. For example, a community psychologist could assist a student in developing preventive and health promotion programs, and a social psychologist with expertise in the area of attitude change could be helpful in planning health education classes. On the university level, students may generate individualized programs that draw upon appropriate courses in nursing, community planning, public administration, medical sociology, biology, economics, health education, and other disciplines. The university health services center may also be enlisted as a training site for program development and evaluation. On the community level, through the development of relationships with health and medical personnel and agencies, curricula can be expanded to include practica in hospitals, clinics, private practices, public health facilities, school health services, and community service organizations (Olbrisch & Sechrest, 1979).

An example of subspecialty training is presented by Ottinger and Roberts (1980) in their description of a postdoctoral practicum in pediatric psychology. The practicum was developed within Purdue's clinical child psychology program and affords the opportunity for advanced students to receive training in pediatric psychology without having to make a commitment to a specialized internship. Initially, a relationship was developed with a community-based pediatrician who referred patients and their families with psychological problems that accompanied physical ailments. The pediatrician, student, and a supervising psychologist would meet regularly to review cases. The pediatrician would assume responsibility for educating the student on medical aspects of each case, and the psychologist and student instructed the pediatrician on psychological factors and treatment modalities. Clients would be seen in the pediatrician's office, in hospitals, and in the university psychological clinic. As the program evolved, students began providing ward consultation and child management consultation to hospital nursing staffs. Soon referrals from other pediatricians were being accepted. One of the pediatricians then began offering a course entitled "Pediatrics for the Clinical Psychologist."

A critical consideration in training psychologists for health care is that, in contrast to physicians and social workers, the psychologist's role in health care settings generally is not clearly defined. Psychologists are relative newcomers to many health care settings. Consequently, they will frequently have to assume an active position in defining and establishing their role. This process will require the successive accomplishment of a series of developmental tasks, such as gaining entry and negotiating job descriptions; developing research, training, and consulting contracts; establishing appropriate workspace; developing credibility; building a resource and information network; delineating a target population; and promoting awareness of their expertise. To prepare psychologists to complete these tasks successfully, training programs will need to convey an understanding of inter- and intraorganizational behavior, the cultural traditions and politics of medical settings, and the expectations of medical personnel regarding psychologists. Additionally, specialized skills will be needed to meet unique demands of the health care environment, such as training physicians and nurses in psychotherapeutic techniques, performing brief assessment and treatment, and functioning as part of a medical team. Chapter 9 of this volume illustrates similar developmental issues with respect to any mental health professional establishing a role in a primary care setting.

Psychiatry

Although psychiatry shares responsibility with other mental health disciplines in training primary health care providers, it is in an especially ideal position to contribute to this effort. Psychiatrists and other primary care physicians share a common medical knowledge base and well-established roles within the health care arena. The family medicine physician shares with the psychiatrist a strong interest in the family. Psychiatrists are more accessible to primary care physicians for consultation in hospitals, since other mental health professionals often have difficulty obtaining hospital admitting privileges. Finally, psychiatrists and primary care physicians have opportunities to establish collaborative relationships through such organizations as local medical associations or faculty appointments in medical schools.

Historically, however, the impact psychiatry has had on the training and practice of primary care physicians has been meager. Until World War II, with only a few notable exceptions, psychiatry was a specialty quite isolated from the mainstream of medical practice (Mental Health and Primary Medical Care, 1980). During World War II psychiatrists and other physicians had the opportunity to work more closely in treating patients. It seemed that after the war's end the integration of psychosocial and biological medicine was close at hand. However, such a biopsychosocial integration ran against the general trend of increased medical specialization (Callen & Davis, 1978). Furthermore, during the postwar period, psychiatry was becoming more involved in the psychoanalytic paradigm, which tended further to split the patient into component parts rather than an integrated biological whole (Mental Health and Primary Medical Care, 1980). Thus, despite numerous efforts to assist in training primary health care providers, psychiatry's impact on other physicians was disappointingly poor during the decades immediately after World War II. The dichotomy between the physical and mental aspects of health persisted (Mental Health and Primary Care, 1980).

The current upsurge of interest in the integration of physical and mental health service delivery offers psychiatry a new opportunity to substantively contribute to the training of its primary care colleagues. Although psychiatrists may offer training in many important aspects of the primary care curriculum, Goldberg (1979) delineates four training areas which he thinks cannot be delegated to other professionals: assessment of physical symptoms that may be psychological in origin, diagnosis of psychiatric conditions that require organic investigations or treatment, use of psychotropic medication, and recognition of conditions needing referral for more specialized psychiatric treatment.

To whatever extent psychiatrists contribute to the training of primary care physicians, there are a number of characteristics which may maximize the effectiveness of their involvement. The Committee on Preventive Psychiatry of the Group for the Advancement of Psychiatry (GAP) suggests that psychiatrists need to be attuned to the inherent limitations of a primary care practice, adept at adapting their educational endeavors to the values inherent in the particular settings in which they teach, and experienced in identifying and demonstrating how psychiatry may be used in a primary care practice (Mental Health and Primary Medical Care, 1980). The GAP Committee also recommends that psychiatrists place more emphasis on the development and functioning of the normal individual than is traditional in their own specialty training. Finally, in order to ensure that psychiatrists are prepared to meet these challenges, GAP suggests that residency programs in psychiatry provide training in consultation-liaison work in a wide range of clinical settings *and* prepare all trainees to teach and practice in primary health care settings (Mental Health and Primary Medical Care, 1980).

Primary Care Medicine

Primary care physicians, including family practitioners, general pediatricians, and general internists, constitute the major subgroup of physicians needing behavioral sciences and mental health skills (Regier & Rosenfeld, 1977). A composite analysis of a number of research efforts in psychiatric epidemiology concludes that the rate of defined mental disorder in primary care populations ranges from 10 to 20 percent (Hankin & Oktay, 1979). Furthermore, this does not include individuals experiencing transient problems of living who also need some assistance. Although serious methodological problems make computations of these rates difficult, rates ranging from 20 to 80 percent are indicative of the key role to be played by primary care physicians (Regier & Rosenfeld, 1977).

For several reasons, people will continue to use primary care physicians for their mental health problems. Visiting one's primary care physician is less stigmatizing than pursuing psychiatric treatment, is often more convenient, is usually reimbursable under most insurance systems, and is frequently based on a long-term, trusting relationship. It has been strongly suggested that this widespread practice even makes good common sense. The advantages of the primary care physician serving as the primary mental health care giver include the ability to maintain a longer-term continuity of care and the greater knowledge and contact the physician may have with all family members. Furthermore, it is argued that it is potentially more efficient for one individual to evaluate and weigh the physical, emotional, and psychosocial aspects of the problem (Tantam, 1979). In order to effectively provide this myriad of services, however, the primary care physician must receive rigorous and relevant training.

Many family practice residency programs are now fairly well grounded in providing their trainees with a behavioral science curriculum component. (For example, see Chapter 11 of this volume.) The Health Professionals Education Assistance Act (PL 94-484) supports the extension of this trend to general pediatrics and internal medicine residencies as well.

Researchers and theoreticians have begun to address the issue of what should be included in the psychosocial curriculum of primary care residency programs. Callen and Davis (1978) asked general physicians practicing in small rural communities to rate the importance of 36 different psychosocial skills in their day-to-day practice of medicine. The highest-ranked items include using psychotropic medication, talking to patients about their emotional problems, treating depression, instituting referral, making a diagnosis, and evaluating suicidal risk. The authors recommended that the 12 top-ranked items receive special emphasis in family practice training programs. A similar study by Fisher and associates (1973) concluded that the most useful training topics are managing milder disorders, skill at interviewing, recognizing disorders, and using psychotropic drugs. Johnson and Snibbe (1975) developed a similar list of mental health topics with which the physician should be familiar.

Marsland and associates (1976) have identified hypertension, headaches, psychosocial and family problems, behavioral disturbances, anxiety, depression, medical noncompliance, and pain as common problems in family practice.

Goldberg (1979) identified a number of interviewing skills, such as asking open-ended questions and taking less control of an interview at the beginning as leading to more accurate detection of mental disorders. He also proposes a format for primary care physicians in assessing a patient's current psychological status.

The report of the NIMH Workgroup on Mental Health Training of Primary Care Providers recommends a number of training priorities: Primary care practitioners should be adept at "diagnosis, should know appropriate indications and dosages of psychotropic drugs, should be familiar with psychodynamics . . . for patient management or therapy, and should have a capacity for facilitating appropriate environmental interventions" (Regier & Rosenfeld, 1977: 15). The workgroup also suggests that the physician needs to cultivate self-knowledge, develop a tolerance and sensitivity toward individuals at risk for mental disorder, recognize a psychiatric emergency, distinguish between various concomitant causes of mental illness, be able to recognize his or her own treatment limits, and be effective in using other mental health specialists as needed. These skills need to be developed in order to serve individuals suffering from (in order of frequency seen in primary care practice) neurotic disorders, psychophysiologic disorders, behavioral disturbances of childhood, character disorders, and more severe depressive and schizophrenic psychotic disorders. In addition, the NIMH workgroup on mental health training endorses more outpatient or ambulatory care training rather than the more traditional inpatient experience (Regier & Rosenfeld, 1977).

In conjunction with curriculum recommendations, preliminary assessments are being undertaken to determine how best to incorporate the necessary skills and knowledge in the training of primary care physicians. One study describes a case presentation-teaching model dealing with recognition and treatment of psychological issues presented by primary care patients (Smarr & Berkow, 1977). Another recounts a method of teaching family dynamics to primary care residents (Guttman & Sigal, 1977). Goldberg et al. (1980) report on a training program designed to maximize the accuracy with which family doctors diagnose psychiatric disturbances. Authier (Chapter 11 of this volume) describes a family life cycle curriculum for training family medicine residents. In addition, a number of other training programs are currently operating which have not yet been documented in books or journal articles. Clearly, a base of program experience is beginning to be established.

Model Training Programs

Each of the disciplines which are necessary in fostering the integration of health and mental health service delivery are at various stages of maximizing their contribution to the effort. Within the limits of the current state of the art, the following two programs are described as a means of demonstrating the wealth of variables which may be called upon in developing a relevant training curriculum.

Community Mental Health for Family Physicians

This training project is designed to upgrade the quality and scope of the psychiatric skills and knowledge of family medicine physicians. The program is a cooperative venture of three organizations. The training of residents and medical students takes place at three different training sites located in the Tampa-St. Petersburg area of Florida. The project is funded by a three-year grant from the National Institute of Mental Health.

The Northside Community Mental Health Center (NCMHC), the Departments of Psychiatry and Family Medicine of the University of South Florida (USF), and Bayfront Medical Center (BMC) developed an affiliation agreement to provide the targeted trainees a thorough and useful behavioral sciences educational experience. The training program is staffed by a faculty member of the USF Department of Psychiatry, a faculty member of the USF Department of Family Medicine, and the Outpatient Program Manager of NCMHC.

Trainees participating in the program are first-, second-, and third-year family medicine residents and senior medical students. The family medicine residents from Bayfront Medical Center are involved as a requirement of their residency program. The USF medical students become involved in the training project by choosing an elective one- or two-month joint rotation in Family Medicine and Psychiatry. The student rotation takes place at Northside and includes involvement in every aspect of the curriculum in which the family medicine residents participate.

The main sites for training are the Northside Community Mental Health Center, the Ambulatory Care Clinic at USF in Tampa, and the Family Practice Clinic at Bayfront Medical Center in St. Petersburg. The Family Medicine residents are required to complete a two-month psychiatry rotation at Northside. In addition, all involved trainees receive weekly case-oriented consultation from a member of the program's behavioral sciences training staff at both the Bayfront Family Practice Clinic and the USF Ambulatory Care Clinic.

The general goals of the full training program are to increase the interviewing, diagnostic, intervention, case management, and primary prevention efforts and abilities of primary care physicians. There are several curriculum components designed to ensure successful completion of these goals and objectives.

Curriculum

There are two major elements of the training curriculum: a two-month psychiatry rotation at Northside and a year-round, on-site consultation service conducted at the Bayfront Medical Center. The Psychiatry rotation includes a number of educational experiences. For example, at Northside the trainee collaboratively conducts a psychotropic medication clinic with the principal Department of Psychiatry faculty member involved in the program. The clinic serves patients who are in psychotherapy with other mental health professionals at Northside but who also need to be evaluated and/or followed up with adjunctive medication.

The trainee also collaboratively conducts a medical consultation clinic with the principal Family Medicine faculty member. The patients served by this clinic are individuals receiving mental health services who also have a suspected or diagnosed medical problem associated with the emotional problem bringing them to Northside. The first task of the trainee is to determine what, if any, treatable physical abnormality may be contributing to the emotional difficulty; second, the trainee works with the Northside staff in providing the comprehensive treatment needed by the patient. As part of this medical consultation clinic the trainee and faculty member give biweekly lectures to the non-medical Northside clinical staff on common medical illnesses associated with various emotional difficulties.

A final clinic in which the trainee participates is the USF Ambulatory Care Clinic. The Family Medicine Clinic at this location is conducted by the trainee and the principal Family Medicine faculty member involved in the program. A major focus of the clinic is to teach the trainee to recognize the emotional aspects of presenting medical problems.

Each trainee rotating through Northside also serves as participant/observer of Northside clinical staff on crisis interviews, intake sessions, and psychotherapy sessions. As the residents become familiar with the procedures of Northside and with the skills and knowledge required to serve the patient population, they are given a small caseload of individuals needing brief psychotherapy treatment. Each of these cases is closely supervised by a Northside clinical staff member.

A series of 13 tutorial seminars is also offered to each of the residents during their rotation. The topics covered and the order in which the tutorials are presented are designed to provide trainees with important basic knowledge which is then used and amplified in other portions of the curriculum. The specific tutorial topics are Psychotropic Medication, Crisis Intervention, Basic Diagnostic Categories, Introduction to Basic Modes of Therapy, Defense Mechanisms, Common Psychiatric Problems in Primary Care, Stress Management, Relaxation Training, Family Dynamics, Community Mental Health, Skills and Roles of Mental Health Professionals, Psychological Testing, and Depression and Suicidal/Homicidal Assessment.

Each of the trainees is also scheduled for night call on the 16-bed Inpatient Psychiatric Unit at Northside. Furthermore, they take time serving as Medical Officer of the Day (M.O.D.) during their outpatient duty hours. The M.O.D. may be called by any Northside staff member when medical consultation or action is needed, such as involuntary commitment or treatment for medication side-effects.

The training program is further augmented by the use of videotaping and one-way mirror observation of interviews. Each trainee videotapes and receives an evaluation on a minimum of two patient interviews. Each trainee is also observed through a one-way mirror by his or her clinical supervisor at Northside in addition to observing interviews conducted by other Northside clinicians.

Weekly USF Department of Psychiatry Adult Clinical Rounds and Child Psychiatry Case Conferences held at Northside are an additional component of the rotation curriculum. Finally, a periodical and book library has been established which is located in the trainee's office to assure ready accessibility.

The second major element of the training program is consultation con-ducted at the affiliate residency site in St. Petersburg. All 20 Bayfront Medical Center Residents receive weekly consultation at the Family Medi-cine Clinic from the Northside outpatient manager. The residents are ob-served interviewing patients and are given feedback on their interviewing style and skills. Also, the consultant periodically interviews selected pa-tients as a means of modeling good interview and intervention skills. The Northside consultant is regularly scheduled for noontime conference presen-tations one day a week.

Informal discussions of theory, practice, and research in the mental health field also occurs when the residents have breaks in their patient schedules. The consultation provided at the outpatient facility in which the residents receive much of their primary care training allows for a natural integration of health and mental health knowledge, in addition to encourag-ing the generalization of recently gained psychiatric skills to their medical practices.

Evaluation

The six-part evaluation package is an important element of this training paradigm. The evaluation assesses the effectiveness of the project, the per-formance level of the trainees, and areas of the curriculum needing manage-ment attention. The six components stress a competency-based formula for evaluation.

The first element in the evaluation package is the Assessment of Psychiat-ric Knowledge, a 40-item objective test administered both before and after the two-month psychiatry rotation. Items for this test are based on the content of the tutorial seminar series and the goals and objectives of the training program.

The second element seeks to evaluate the trainee's interview skills. At the beginning and end of the rotation, the trainee videotapes a patient interview, which is evaluated by skilled clinicians according to a prepared rating scale. Another similar exercise is used to evaluate the trainee's observation skills. Again, at the beginning and end of the rotation, the trainee watches a videotaped patient interview conducted by an experienced clinician. The trainee then indicates his or her observations on a form which basically follows a mental status format.

Two additional components of the evaluative package are the supervisor's evaluation of the trainee and the trainee's evaluation of the rotation. Finally, each trainee completes a daily activity log which is designed to capture each portion of the curriculum in which the trainee actually participates.

The results of each of the evaluation components is not only used at the end of a rotation or at the end of a year to determine the effectiveness of the program, but is monitored throughout each rotation to ensure that the trainee is afforded the opportunity to gain maximum benefit from the training experience.

The Houston Consortium Training Program

In 1976, an interagency and interinstitutional consortium was formed in Houston, Texas, to provide primary care-mental health training. In 1977, it received a three-year NIMH grant award. The participating educational institutions include Baylor College of Medicine (Departments of Psychiatry, Community Medicine, Internal Medicine, and Pediatrics); the University of Texas Health Science Center at the Houston School of Nursing; and the University of Houston Graduate School of Social Work. The service agencies cooperating in this educational project include the Harris County Hospital District and the Mental Health/Mental Retardation Authority of Harris County (Moffic, Cheney, Adams, Chacko, Tristan, & Gomez, 1979).

The project's practicum training site is the Casa de Amigos Neighborhood Health Center, which serves a predominantly low-income Mexican and black community. This site was chosen because it housed a child and adult primary health care agency as well as a mental health center. In addition, a number of trainees of the educational institutions involved in the consortium were already receiving practicum training at this site. The didactic portion of the training project is provided at Baylor's Department of Psychiatry (Moffic et al., 1979).

The objectives of the training consortium are (1) to educate mental health trainees in the delivery of mental health services, both as members of primary care teams and secondary mental health teams; (2) to enable primary care professionals and trainees to acquire mental health skills that will help them to better serve their patients; (3) to provide health (including mental health) caregivers with cross-cultural and psychosocial perspectives in the delivery of care to minority populations; and (4) to develop team and interdisciplinary working skills in the delivery of health and mental health services in primary care settings (Adams, Brochstein, Cheney, Friese, & Tristan, 1978).

The trainees benefiting from the educational program include internal medicine residents, pediatric residents, medical students, graduate social work students, and psychiatric nursing students. All of these trainees are placed on integrated primary care teams. The social work trainees provide mental health assessment and services for patients and assist the primary care team in addressing mental health issues. Fourth-year psychiatry residents and clinical psychology interns are members of a secondary mental health team that provides consultation and backup to the primary care teams (Moffic et al., 1979).

Curriculum

Trainees from each of the disciplines represented in the consortium participate in activities typical of any practicum placement for that group. For example, the residents and medical students run clinics in the primary care health clinic, the social work graduate students render psychosocial assessment and psychotherapeutic services, the psychiatry residents provide psychiatric evaluations and treatment, and the psychology interns conduct psychological assessments and psychotherapy. Each group also receives separate supervision and training from faculty in its respective discipline.

The design of the program seeks to encourage interdisciplinary teaching and sharing of perceptions, skills, and information through several aspects of the curriculum. First, the primary care team, comprised of physician and social work trainees, is an organizational method that encourages close interaction. In addition, the secondary mental health trainee team is located in close physical proximity to the primary health care team. Also, the program includes a generic interdisciplinary mental health didactic curriculum for all primary care and mental health trainees. The didactic presentations that are useful to all trainees are scheduled and jointly presented to all trainees. Finally, consortium trainees and faculty cooperatively participate in case presentations and site visits to community service organizations.

Although interdisciplinary pursuits are encouraged by the consortium, as the training program developed it became necessary to allow for the development of disciplinary orthodoxy as well. Thus, the trainees are involved in separate didactic case presentation and trainee-faculty conferences according to discipline.

Evaluation

The formal evaluation process includes the assessment of consortium developments through time, measurement of trainees' cognitive gains, measurement of trainee attitudinal change, and the analysis of the process of service delivery provided to patients of the health center (Moffic et al., 1979). Trainee cognitive and attitudinal changes are measured by paper-and-pencil objective tests. The assessment of consortium developments through time and a description of the project are summarized in several articles appearing in the *International Journal of Mental Health* (1979).

Future Directions in Training

Initiatives in the areas of service and research during the 1970s have resulted in a professional manpower strategy emphasizing the integration of physical and mental health services. The focus during the current decade must be on the response that the professional training programs will make to these new directions. At this time, a comprehensive approach to training professionals in integrated health services is clearly in a formative stage of development.

The disciplines involved in this major undertaking have, to varying extents, defined a range of roles they may assume and have begun, in part, to prepare their trainees for such roles. Professional organizations such as the American Psychological Association, the National Association of Social Work, and the American Psychiatric Association have stepped up their efforts in addressing health-mental health care issues. Some university training programs are responding by merely emphasizing the importance of health-mental health integration, while others are adding special components to the curriculum and some are even developing entirely new and innovative educational projects. Nonetheless, substantial effort must continue in research, planning, and evaluation of current and future training programs in order to assure the establishment of a potent nationwide training effort.

In the areas of research, Burns and her colleagues (1979) delineated a number of topics which require further exploration: the prevalence of mental disorder in primary health care settings, the outcomes of mental health services provided by the primary health care sector, the needs of special populations seen by primary care physicians, and the financing and cost of services.

Evaluation for current training programs in formative as well as summative aspects is another task which must be tackled. Formative evaluation should include the assessment of knowledge and skill acquisition during graduate training and postdoctoral internships and residencies. Specific recommendations should be made concerning the optimum faculty mixture, the most effective teaching and practice aides, the manner in which organizational structure may positively affect training efforts, and what program characteristics are most highly valued and rated by the trainees.

Summative or "bottom line" evaluation must address a number of equally important issues. First, how do the programs influence the trainees after completion of their postgraduate education? For example, do more psychologists and social workers choose to work in primary health care settings? Do primary care physicians, once they are in practice, feel more comfortable and knowledgeable about their patients' emotional distress? How effective are the primary care physicians in administering to the mental health needs of their patients? And finally, are graduates of the special mental health training programs viewed by practicing primary care physicians as more helpful and knowledgeable than mental health professionals not receiving the specialized training?

As the results of research endeavors and program evaluations surface, appropriate modifications must be made in developing and planning future educational efforts. Hence, the training of professionals for health-mental health integration will continue to become more relevant and effective.

References

Adams, G. L., & Cheney, C. C. Introduction. *International Journal of Mental Health,* 1979, 8, 3-5.

Adams, G. L., Brochstein, J. R., Cheney, C. C., Friese, J. H., & Tristan, M. P. A primary care/mental health training and service model. *American Journal of Psychiatry,* 1978, 135, 121-123.

Bibace, R., & Walsh, M. E. Clinical developmental psychologists in family practice settings. *Professional Psychology,* 1979, 10, 441-450.

Bloom, L. S. Psychology and cardiology: Collaboration in coronary treatment and prevention. *Professional Psychology,* 1979, 10, 485-490.

Brown, B. S., & Regier, D. A. How NIMH now views the primary care practitioner. *Practical Psychology for Physicians,* 1977, 4, 12-14.

Budman, S. H., & Clifford, M. Short-term group therapy for couples in a health maintenance organization. *Professional Psychology,* 1979, 10, 419-429.

Burns, B. J., Regier, D. A., Goldberg, I. D., & Kessler, L. G. Future directions in primary care/mental health research. *International Journal of Mental Health,* 1979, 8, 130-140.

Cain, L. P. Preparing a psychotic patient for major surgery. *Social Casework,* 1974, 55, 401-408.

Callen, K. E., & Davis, D. The general practitioner: How much psychiatric education? *Psychosomatics,* 1978, 19, 409-413.

Falck, H. S. Social work in health settings. *Social Work in Health Care,* 1978, 3, 395-403.

Fisher, J. V., Fowler, H., & Fabrega, H. Family physicians want more postgraduate psychiatric training. *Patient Care,* 1973, 7, 54-57.

Goldberg, D. Detection and assessment of emotional disorders in a primary care setting. *International Journal of Mental Health,* 1979, 8, 30-48.

Goldberg, D., Steele, J. J., Smith, C., & Spivey, L. Training family doctors to recognize psychiatric illness with increased accuracy. *The Lancet,* 1980, September, 521-523.

Goldberg, R. L. The social worker and the family physician. *Social Casework,* 1973, 54, 489-495.

Grzesiak, R. C. Psychological services in rehabilitation medicine: Clinical aspects of rehabilitation psychology. *Professional Psychology,* 1979, 10, 511-520.

Guttman, H. A., & Sigal, J. J. Teaching family psychodynamics in a family practice center: One experience. *International Journal of Psychiatry in Medicine,* 1977, 8, 383-392.

Hanna, E. A., & Schachter, J. G. An integration of psycho-social concepts into the education of general practitioners. *Social Work in Health Care,* 1979, 4, 393-408.

Hankin, J., & Oktay, J. *Mental disorder and primary medical care: An analytical review of the literature.* NIMH Monograph Series D, No. 5. DHEW Publication No. (ADM) 78-661. Washington, DC: Government Printing Office, 1979.

Health Professions Educational Assistance Act of 1976. Public Law 94-484, October 20, 1976.

Institute of Medicine. A conference report, volume 1, *Mental health services in general health care.* Washington, DC: National Academy of Sciences, 1979.

Johnson, W., & Snibbe, J. The selection of a psychiatric curriculum for medical students: Results of a survey. *American Journal of Psychiatry,* 1975, 132, 513-516.

Kerson, T. S. Sixty years ago: Hospital social work in 1918. *Social Work in Health Care,* 1979, 4, 331-343.

Korpela, J. W. Social work assistance in private pediatric practice. *Social Casework,* 1973, 54, 537-544.

Kumabe, K., Nishida, C., O'Hara, D., & Woodruff, C. *A handbook for social work education and practice in community health settings.* Honolulu: University of Hawaii School of Social Work, 1977.

Lebray, P. R. Geropsychology in long-term care settings. *Professional Psychology,* 1979, 10, 475-484.

Marsland, A. H., Wood, M. B., & Mayo, F. The databank of patient care, curriculum and research in family practice: 526,196 patient problems. *Journal of Family Practice,* 1976, 3, 25-28.

Mental Health and Primary Medical Care. Committee on Preventive Psychiatry, Group for the Advancement of Psychiatry. New York: Mental Health Materials Center, 1980.

Mental Health Systems Act of 1980. Public Law 96-398, October 7, 1980.

Moffic, H. S., Cheney, C. C., Adams, G. L., Chacko, R. C., Tristan, M. P., & Gomez, E. A. Mental health, the poor, and the promised land—The Houston Consortium training program. *International Journal of Mental Health,* 1979, 8, 74-88.

Morse, J. Family involvement in pediatric dialysis and transplantation. *Social Casework,* 1974, 55, 216-223.

Nieman, D. A., & Hoops, A. Can private hospitals afford to provide social services? *Social Work in Health Care,* 1977, 3, 175-180.

Olbrisch, M. E., & Sechrest, L. Educating health psychologists in traditional graduate training programs. *Professional Psychology,* 1979, 10, 589-595.

Ottinger, D. R., & Roberts, M. C. A university-based predoctoral practicum in pediatric psychology. *Professional Psychology,* 1980, 11, 707-713.

Regier, D. A., Goldberg, I. D., & Taube, C. A. The de facto U.S. mental health services system: A public health perspective. *Archives of General Psychiatry,* 1978, 35, 685-693.

Regier, D. A., & Rosenfeld, A. H. The report of the NIMH workshop on mental health training of primary care providers. Washington, DC: National Institute of Mental Health, 1977.

Sachs, R. H. Psychology and dentistry. *Professional Psychology,* 1979, 10, 521-528.

Smarr, E. R., & Berkow, M. D. Teaching psychological medicine to family practice residents. *American Journal of Psychiatry,* 1977, 134, 984-987.

Sokol, B. The clinical social worker as a member of a health team in a coronary care unit. *Clinical Social Work Journal,* 1976, 4, 269-275.

Stone, G. C. A specialized doctoral program in health psychology: Considerations in its evolution. *Professional Psychology,* 1979, 10, 596-604.

Tantam, D. Primary mental health care in the United Kingdom. *International Journal of Mental Health,* 1979, 8, 108-129.

White, S. L. The impact of mental health services on medical care utilization: Economic and organizational implications. *Hospital & Community Psychiatry,* 1981, 32, 311-319.

World Health Organization. *Psychiatry and primary medical care.* Copenhagen: Regional Office for Europe, 1973.

Wright, L. A comprehensive program for mental health and behavioral medicine in a large children's hospital. *Professional Psychology,* 1979, 10, 458-466.

11

Integrated Medical Training

A Family Focus

Jerry Authier
University of Nebraska Medical Center

Family medicine educators and other primary care specialists emphasize primary care medicine as one level of care which requires an integration of health and mental health skills and knowledge. The need for such an integration becomes obvious when one considers that many investigations have demonstrated that 50 percent or more of the problems presented to a primary care physician have a psychological component. For example, Carmichael (1978), a noted authority in the field of family medicine, indicates that in "more than 80% of encounters in family practice the problems involve self limited illnesses, prevention, or psychosocial difficulties." Young (1978) claims that approximately 50 percent of ambulatory medical patients suffer from psychosocial problems. He further claims that about 45 percent require psychotherapeutic or supportive care within the context of family medical practice, while only five percent require intervention by mental health professionals. Therefore, the need for training on the psychosocial aspects of health to specialists in the field of family medicine is paramount.

Authorities in the field of family medicine have stressed the need for an integrated health and mental health care delivery system by advocating the inclusion of behavioral sciences in the curriculum of family medicine. The Willard Report (1968), which provided the primary guidelines for education

AUTHOR'S NOTE: I wish to acknowledge my team members from the Section of Family Behavior, William B. Long, Evelyn R. Alperin, Jacque Krier, and Gerald Pierce. Moreover, thanks are extended to the other Department of Family Practice staff members, especially Acting Chairperson Margaret Faithe, for their support and encouragement in the implementation of the Family Behavioral Training. Finally, a special note of thanks to Kathy McCallan and Jan Church for assistance that extended beyond that of secretaries.

in family practice, emphasized the need for a behavioral science focus as part of the training of family physicians. The report stated:

> These disciplines (e.g., sociology, social psychology, and anthropology) should help the student acquire a holistic approach to health and disease and to recognize the interrelationships of cultural, social, psychologic, and environmental factors with the physiologic and biochemical processes of the body. They should help the student to understand his/her own behavior better and that of many of his/her associates and patients and how each may affect the other and the response to therapy by the patient. These disciplines should provide other useful content including an understanding of the variable roles of family members in different cultures; the causes and processes of family disorganization and its effects upon the family members; social structure; social roles and role conflicts; value systems; medicine, religion, and law as social institutions and their interrelationship in historic context; and an understanding of the communication process for interviewing and counseling [p. 258].

Geyman (1971) also stated that the component disciplines of the behavioral sciences can add to the understanding of the individual and the family.

Because of the need to recognize and treat the large number of psychosocial problems that are presented to physicians, the teaching of behavioral sciences within family practice training programs will presumably lead to more comprehensive care and a better integration of health and mental health services. Before describing how behavioral training is incorporated into the University of Nebraska Family Practice Residency Training Program, the following section will explore the philosophical underpinnings of treatment of individuals within the family context.

Family-Focused Medicine

For more than a decade, family medicine educators have been stressing the need for training residents in the understanding of family dynamics as a means of providing them with the knowledge necessary to treat the individual within the context of his or her family. Geyman (1971), for example, concluded that "family practice programs should give future family physicians the training they need for early diagnosis, prevention and treatment of common emotional problems in the family" (p. 155). Schmidt (1978) summarizes the basis for such an emphasis when he outlines the family's contribution to the cure of the disease, the family's response to chronic disease, and the family's desire or need for family-oriented care as three major reasons for the family physician to consider the family in the provision of treatment.

Bauman and Grace (1977) underscore the family's contribution to the cause of the disease as the primary reason for the need for a family-focused approach to the delivery of integrated health care.

> The physician who is on the front lines of continuous medical care of the people in the community can redefine the problems seen in an individual as being manifestations of a disturbance in the patient's family unit. The basis for this concept is that the person who is ill is often the symptom carrier for the whole family and thus acts as a signal that the entire family relationship is in distress [p. 1135].

A review of research in this area (Schmidt, 1978) provides evidence that a family-focused approach enhances diagnosis and treatment within both health and mental health settings. Authier, Starr, and Authier (1979) suggest that family-focused medicine can simplify the diagnosis and then the treatment of many problems. They indicate that patterns and dynamics present in families have significant implications for medical diagnosis and treatment. When physicians overlook information regarding the family system, they may arrive at erroneous conclusions about the nature of the illness and treatment needed. Treatment approaches which ignore the family of the patient run the risk of being sabotaged or thwarted by the family system. This latter point is echoed by Jaffe (1978), who states that the family is the most important external force shaping the individual's personality, emotional difficulties, and the expression of physical illness. Therefore, family therapy, in addition to other approaches to physical illness, may be a key factor in successful treatment.

Another function of the family is to help family physicians provide health maintenance and primary prevention. The role of the family with regard to maintaining the interpersonal, psychological, and emotional health and functioning of the individual is generally more apparent than is its role with regard to maintaining physical health. Still, few would deny that teaching health behaviors, be they psychological or physical, is a family task and that family patterns and organization have a great impact on health and disease processes.

Authorities in the field of family medicine recognize the importance of the family with regard to health maintenance issues. For example, Bauman and Grace (1977) indicate that the family physician "is in an advantageous position to intervene at an early stage in the development of pathological family processes, thus frequently preventing long-term psychiatric therapy and/or psychosomatic concomitants" (p. 24). They claim it is necessary for the family physician to view the "patient" as the symptom carrier for the whole family. Thus, the "healthy" members of the family may sustain or precipitate the problem in the symptomatic member. If a family physician can talk periodically with the family and help them to express their feelings, prevention of destructive actions, feelings and even morbidity can occur. Though not specifically dealing with health maintenance, case examples by Bursten (1964) and Shoemaker et al. (1977) demonstrate that a family physician can intervene, even after the fact, to bring about more appropriate health behavior within the family system. Bursten's (1964) case demonstrates how a family conflict resulted in the husband, with mild chronic bronchitis, assuming the role of a sick and complaining patient rather than becoming more assertive with his domineering wife.

Given that the family is responsible for teaching health behavior to its respective members, and that the family is the treatment unit of family medicine, it is paramount that the family orientation become a part of health maintenance education. This seems particularly important since a recent study by Lewis (1976) which demonstrates that certain family characteristics are associated with low rates of physical illness. The author concluded that there

> does appear to be something about the way a family is organized that may influence the vulnerability of the family members to illness. This adds weight to the writings of those clinicians and investigators who have suggested that an adequate model of disease must attend not only to the individual but consider also the family as a possible unit of illness [p. 48].

In spite of the above points, there is still considerable resistance among residents in family practice training programs to accept the concept of the individual within the context of the family as a major component that makes their specialty distinctive from the other primary or secondary medical specialties. The resistance appears to stem largely from the fact that throughout their training medical students are exposed for the most part to a medical, biological, or disease model rather than to an individual or family model or treatment. As a consequence, they adopt an attitude that the medical model is the only appropriate model for them as physicians. Family medicine educators have the task of changing this attitude.

Family Behavioral Training

The Department of Family Practice at the University of Nebraska includes a Section of Family Behavior. This section maintains the primary goal of helping family practice residents treat the psychobiosocial problems of the family by emphasizing an understanding of the family, teaching interpersonal and/or counseling skills of the resident, and teaching the diagnosis and treatment of psychobiosocial dysfunctions. This goal is carried out primarily through a team effort. The team consists of a psychiatrist, who was formerly a family physician, a clinical psychologist, and three social workers. Such a team approach allows for a broad emphasis, encompassing the expertise of various authorities in the field.

The Family Practice Residency Training Program consists of a three-year sequence. Accordingly, the Family Behavior Team attempts to offer instruction tailored to the year level of the resident. First-year house officers are taught how to form an effective doctor/patient relationship and manage patients with fairly routine medical problems. This is accomplished mainly through the review of ten videotaped doctor/patient interactions and ten behavioral science grand rounds. During the second year, the focus shifts to the family. A series of didactic seminars explores the family life cycle as a means for understanding and diagnosing individual problems within a family context. In this year emphasis is also placed on counseling, including family behavioral and dynamic counseling and brief therapy skills to enhance the resident's ability to intervene when a patient is suffering from one of the psychobiosocial dysfunctions. The combined family and psychobiosocial dysfunction emphasis is continued throughout the third year by means of eight videotaped review sessions. Various "hallway" consultations, co-therapy when treating family or individual patient (i.e., a resident and a Family Behavior Team member), and additional grand round topics are offered throughout the residency as a means of integrating health and mental health issues within the context of the training program.

In conjunction with the above, our residents are also offered a one-month Family Practice Orientation. Here they are assigned families and required to chart family problems, including a family tree, and are exposed to the other aspects of training which have a family focus. This orientation process promotes the attitude change from the disease/medical model to the family medical model. It is hoped that, as a consequence of this training, our family physicians will begin to question the impact that a presenting problem, no matter how purely physical it may seem, may be having on the health and well-being of other family members.

Although various modalities are used to emphasize the relationship between health and mental health in the family, the Family Life Cycle Seminars are perhaps the main training tools for accomplishing this goal.

The Family Life Cycle Seminars

As a conceptual framework, the family life cycle "can be useful to the
family physician in everyday practice by increasing his/her awareness of
potential crisis in the individual patient and his/her family" (Geyman, 1977:
573). Although there are several ways of dealing with the life cycle, the
schema developed by Hill (1958) and elaborated upon by Authier (1979)
seems most relevant to the practice of family medicine. This schema divides
family life into four potential crisis periods, outlined in Table 11.1.

Before examining each of these crisis periods, several seminars are discussed which examine more general issues of family structure and dynamics. Throughout there is an emphasis on practical knowledge and skills,
since these are areas in which family physicians look to behavioral scientists
for assistance (Aluise, 1977).

Family Structure

Case examples and various articles are presented during the two seminars
on family dynamics and family communication. For example, one article
demonstrates that the mother commonly functions in the role of family
diagnostician. The residents are cautioned that she may be inclined to give a
problem a name quickly, often a medical term, and in so doing possibly
presses the physician to agree with her specific diagnosis, perhaps to the
degree of compromising the physician's own medical judgment. Other typical health-seeking roles and family dynamics, like the possibility of a sick
member being scapegoated by the family, are stressed. These initial seminars provide the resident with an awareness of the potential of family dynamics in health-seeking behavior so they can effectively intervene while
not playing into what might be malfunctioning family system.

The developmental stages emphasized during the initial Family Life
Cycle Seminars provide the residents with knowledge of courtship, sexuality, and how the new baby can have a potentially disruptive effect on the
family. Certain childhood and adolescent adjustment problems are discussed, such as parents adapting to the struggle for independence among
adolescents. This struggle sometimes results in the parents claiming the
youth is "sick." Or the adolescent may come in claiming to be "sick." The
seminars provide the residents with knowledge which allows them to look

TABLE 11.1   The Family Life Cycle: A Theoretical Framework for Family
Practice Residents

Section I.   Family Structure
A. History and current status of the family in the United States
B. Family dynamics
1. Systems theory
2. Communication theory
C. Developmental aspects of infancy, childhood, and adolescence

Section II.   Crises of Addition
A. The genesis of the family
1. Courtship and premarital counseling
2. Problems of newlyweds (i.e., sexuality)
3. Family planning
4. Problems of pregnancy and a new member of the family (infant)
B. Problems encountered with other new members
1. Stepparent and/or children
2. Child member moving back home
3. Grandparent or parents being added (or aunts, uncles, or other
significant persons)

Section III.   Crises of Demoralization
A. Emotional and behavioral problems of infancy and childhood
1. Mental retardation
2. Minimal brain dysfunction and/or other learning disabilities
B. Emotional and behavioral problems of adolescence
1. Transient situational disturbances
2. Developmental problems
C. Emotional and behavioral problems of adulthood
1. Neuroses
2. Psychoses
3. Personality and other miscellaneous disorders

Section IV.   Crises of Status Shift
A. Move to new community
B. Promotion or demotion
C. Middle years
D. Retirement and late life

Section V.   Crises of Attrition
A. Member(s) moving out
B. Death or significant role loss through illness
C. Divorce

Section VI.   Summary and Treatment
A. Family therapy for the family physician
B. Brief therapeutic techniques for the family physician

for these developmental stages as possible contributory factors to presenting problems in the office, as well as skills in patient education and/or family intervention.

If the resident should determine that developmental crises are contributing to a presenting problem, then intervention through parent education during routine visits is one means of helping the family with its health maintenance task. For illustrative purposes, examples of content provided under each crisis outlined in Table 11.1 will be presented.

Crises of Addition

Topics covered in this portion of the seminar deal with the effect of creating a family and adding new members to it. One of the most vivid examples of such an approach occurs during the initial well-baby check. The family physician has had the advantage of seeing the family as a unit during the course of hospitalization for labor and delivery and has been able to access family dynamics, communication, and how health behavior and emotions are exhibited in the family. With this as a backdrop, the resident can raise questions as to how other family members, especially the father and the youngest child, are adapting to the new addition. Such a "minor crisis" might lead to the husband withdrawing or acting out, sibling rivalry manifested in discipline or school problems, or the wife withdrawing because she no longer feels as much a part of the family since devoting all of her time making certain that the new member is a healthy one.

The resident, through interviewing techniques taught in another segment of training, is able to determine whether or not some of the behaviors being manifested are symptoms of this particular family crisis. If this should be the case, armed with the information from the didactic portions of the seminars, the resident is able to conduct patient education to prevent a major crisis from occurring. If simple patient education is not enough, family intervention in the form of brief family therapy might be necessary. Here the residents are advised to either refer or involve one of the Family Behavior Team staff, since at this point in their training they do not have the skills to provide brief, crisis intervention family therapy. However, they are informed that after they master the family therapy training sessions offered as the last content area of the Family Life Cycle Seminar program, such intervention by them would be appropriate.

Such family intervention represents the practice of health maintenance at the ground level, especially as it applies to mental health issues. Before the new addition to the family begins to develop any kind of "psychiatric" disturbance, the physician, through family-oriented interventions, can guide the family to more appropriate means of coping with stress, improved communication, clarification of roles and expectations, and so forth.

Crises of Demoralization

This segment of the seminar deals with numbers of crises which have the potential to demoralize the family. Essentially, this section covers various psychiatric syndromes. However, it also includes physical conditions that can have psychological consequences, such as paralysis. Having already experienced the disruptive effects of a sick family member, the family physician can provide the necessary mental health services.

For example, one seminar session concerns a young family member with agoraphobia, possibly caused and perpetuated by the family system. Using a videotaped interaction of the family members, the case is discussed with respect to how the family physician can intervene to help the family behave in a manner which would not foster and maintain the phobic condition. The resident involved in the case proceeded to make comments along these lines as he worked with the family. He was effective to the degree that the patient was eventually able to leave the house and was, in fact, looking for work.

Chronic or serious medical illness is still another crisis which has the potential for family demoralization. For example, a family member can become partially paralyzed with a severe cardiac condition. The family is demoralized in two respects; the ill member may die, and role changes are required to accommodate for the disabled family member. Residents are taught that it is necessary for the individual patient to work through these fears and role concerns within the context of the family as a means of enabling both the individual and the family to adjust to the loss of role function.

It is in health problems such as the above that integration of health and mental health services is paramount. This integration is especially necessary if the illness requires some hospitalization or surgical intervention. In such cases there is a need to provide care for the physical problem coupled with supportive counseling for both the individual and the family with respect to the psychological consequences.

Crises of Status Shift

Job changes, moving, and aging are examples of life events that may involve a change in status. One of the seminars in this section involves discussion of the effect one family member undergoing midlife crisis was having on the other members of the family. In essence, the father exhibited depressive symptomatology, causing considerable disturbance within the family system since he was no longer an active and hard-working member. The wife had to assume a more dominant role with which she felt uncomfortable. The wife and husband were seen together as a means of helping him reduce his depressive symptomatology and resume his former role within the family system. The family physician is in a particularly good position to anticipate such a crisis in the middle years and therefore to prevent serious psychological dysfunctions. Since they know their patients and their patients' family systems, they can anticipate whether the 40th or 45th birthday is going to be the one which will cause their patient to have significant adjustment problems. Furthermore, if the physician has an awareness of other environmental factors affecting the family, such as job changes, he or she can anticipate the potential effect a major status shift might have. Anticipatory guidance with respect to how the predictable life crisis is likely to develop and eventually end is another intervention possibility.

Crises of Attrition

The final type of crisis experienced by the family is that of attrition. For example, it is important for the physician to pay careful attention to the family who has a terminally ill member. A family prepared for the loss will not be as disrupted by it. In such cases, the family physician helps the family to maintain its homeostasis, thereby providing preventive treatment. This example illustrates for the resident that the treatment of the family involves the maintenance of family homeostasis.

Family Intervention

Family interventions are important and practical ways to integrate health and mental health care. While the main emphasis in our program is on the use of behavioral techniques, training is also available in dynamic therapy.

Family Behavioral Counseling

Each resident receives a detailed outline of the issues to be addressed once he or she has decided that family intervention is necessary. These issues are outlined in Appendix A. It is hoped that the outline will be a practical heuristic to enable residents to treat families within the time constraints of a busy family practice.

The residents are further instructed that if they feel the resistance to treatment is too great, or if the family chooses to be referred, there are useful things that the family physician can do to assure that the family gets into family therapy with a competent mental health professional. One of the most useful techniques taught is to schedule the appointment with the mental health professional while the family is present. In this way, the physician's relationship with the family is utilized to increase the family's commitment to follow through. Another useful technique is to ask the family to call following their first scheduled appointment. By doing this, the family knows that the physician is interested and is going to monitor their progress. Moreover, residents are instructed to support and encourage the family in their efforts in family therapy each time they see them in the office for other problems. The resident is instructed that once the family discontinues seeing the mental health specialist, it is the family physician who continues to monitor their progress and reinforce those changes in the family system that are in their best interest. If some regression within the family is noted, residents are instructed to bring this to the family's attention. The resident can then work with them directly or again make a referral to a mental health professional.

Family Dynamic Therapy

Residents are given the opportunity to learn what we call "family dynamic therapy" if they have the interest, time, and competency. Competency, for the most part, requires a more thorough understanding of family dynamics. These residents are required to gain a working knowledge of at least one of the major models of family therapy, such as those proposed by Whitaker (1958), Satir (1964), Minuchin (1970), or Haley (1971). Additionally, a brief outline, presented in Appendix B, is given to them as a guide if they decide to use family dynamic therapy.

It is not suggested that family physicians become family therapists. Along these lines, there is agreement with Stephens's (1974) conclusion that

the issue is not whether the theory and practice of family therapy should be an important component of the education of the family physician, but whether his education should be limited to that. Such limitation would be a confusion of whole and part. "Family Medicine" should be preserved as an essentially synonymous but alternative term to "family practice" and should not be appropriated as a synonym for family therapy—a field that has already developed as an independent branch of the tree of knowledge [p. 3].

However, in some instances, not providing family counseling for a family would be a disservice to the family and to the specialty. Since family practice is not limited by organ system, age group, or the area of technical skill, it is incumbent upon the family physican to diagnose and/or treat families in "disease." By doing this, our residents will be practicing an integrated health care model which will help them to become family physicians in the truest sense.

Psychobiosocial Medicine

There are times when it is appropriate for a family physician to focus on the individual suffering from what is traditionally considered a "psychiatric" syndrome. To deal with such patients our residents are taught how to diagnose, manage, and treat those with individual psychopathology.

Interpersonal communication skills are paramount in dealing with the individual who has a psychiatric disturbance. The physician must establish an effective relationship with the patient in order to gather information for a diagnosis and to facilitate treatment. Our program attempts to train such interpersonal skills through a training program entitled "Enriching Intimacy." The goal is to teach the resident those interpersonal skills that are behavioral components of the more global therapeutic characteristics of empathy, respect, and genuineness (Rogers, 1951, Truax & Carkhuff, 1967). The program uses a behavioral approach to teaching relationship skills (Authier & Gustafson, 1973). It draws heavily from microcounseling interview training techniques (Ivey, 1971; Ivey & Authier, 1978).

The residents are required to complete ten videotape reviews during their first year and eight reviews during their second and third years, respectively. These reviews consist of fairly routine office visit procedures during the first year, focusing on basic interviewing and interpersonal skills. The residents are trained to take a medical history, to make the transition from the history to the physical examination, and to terminate an interview. They are also shown how to use various interpersonal skills, such as reflecting a patient's feelings, paraphrasing, and encouraging the patient to talk about difficulties.

The second and third years focus more on traditional "psychiatric" and/or difficult patients, such as the tearfully depressed patient. These review sessions concentrate on helping the resident make the appropriate diagnosis and psychotherapeutic intervention. Therapeutic techniques employed range from brief ventilative, supportive therapy for a grief reaction to brief goal-directed therapy for someone who is suffering from a personality disorder. Additionally, if medications are warranted, the resident is taught to provide appropriate information to the patient regarding the expected results of possible side-effects. How the physician manages drug side-effects is also part of the review. If necessary, one of the Family Behavior Section personnel—usually the psychiatrist or the clinical psychologist—will work with the resident in the capacity of a co-therapist. However, the family behavior specialist tries to maintain the resident in the role of the primary care provider so that the resident can learn to manage difficult patients independently.

Evaluation of Family Behavioral Training

The focus on the individual within the context of his or her family and the practice of psychobiosocial medicine are constantly emphasized during the residents' training. This emphasis should allow the residents to experience an attitudinal change regarding family-focused medicine. Indeed, they appear to be moving from a disease-oriented model to one which focuses on the individual within their family context. This shift is necessary for them to practice family medicine in the manner that makes them family physicians in the truest sense.

Subjective impressions indicate that residents are considering the impact of the patient's family on the patient's presenting problems and are practicing psychobiosocial medicine to a greater extent. Evaluations of the program have been initiated to assess whether the subjective impressions of positive change are valid and significant. It is hoped that the results of these studies will form the basis for future reports documenting the effectiveness of training physicians for integrated family practice.

Appendix A
Guide to Family Behavioral Counseling

I. Offer treatment but inform family of time limit, your competency, and how seeing someone else might be of greater benefit and may even be necessary later.
II. How to get other family members involved.
 A. Solicit their help in treating "X."
 B. Talk about enhancing the family.
 C. Find significant others in family as allies.
 D. Find means of coercing them to come in for treatment.
III. How to treat the family with brief evaluative therapy once family members are involved.
 A. Focus on positive aspects first (e.g., big step for them to come in; have essentially a good family, etc.).

B. Three evaluative phases:
1. Begin first session with the question, "How do each of you *feel* about being here?"
   a. Observe sitting arrangement.
   b. Observe who talks first.
   c. Observe who is most silent.
   d. Observe other nonverbal cues.
      (1) Do they look at each other when they talk?
      (2) Is there anger, hurt, sadness, resentment, or another feeling tone in their voices?
   e. Observe whether they use feeling words to specific questions.
   f. Once they have all admitted to some discomfort, or you've been able to point that out, terminate, with homework assignment—to think of one situation which makes them feel a specific discomfort.
   g. Warn of "flight into health" tendency and encourage them to come back in.
   h. If they don't admit to discomfort, then either terminate or suggest referral, because it looks like they aren't willing to work on enhancing the family.
2. Begin second evaluation session with the question, "How well did each of you do with the homework assignment?"
   a. Which member sabotaged it, if any?
   b. Continue to observe dynamics and verbal and nonverbal cues.
   c. If homework not completed, confront about whether they really want treatment and if they don't terminate.
   d. If homework completed, then facilitate communication regarding trade-off for next week (e.g., She'll not nag about his not coming home right after work if he'll help put the kids to bed at night, OR if he likes to stay at the office two hours, when she would like him home after one, perhaps an agreement of that nature.) When children age 5 or older are involved, they also trade off with each parent. You may need to take additional session(s) to take care of each child due to time constraints of a family physician's practice. Sometimes a family group goal can be reached, and such a family project is helpful (e.g., they all help mom with dishes if she won't complain about this or that responsibility). It is important in these trade-offs to:
      (1) Allow each person to choose what he/she wants the other person to work on (i.e., do or not do). Sometimes working on doing something positive in a particularly difficult family is a better place to start.
      (2) Be specific about the behavior, the time, the place, and, if necessary, how it is to be done.
3. Begin third evaluation session with an assessment of the family's specific homework assignments or trade-offs by asking the question, "How well did each of you do with your specific assignments?"

a. Who sabotaged the homework?

b. Observe verbal and nonverbal cues. (Who's blaming whom and how is this being manifested?)

c. If children involved, is there a white knight or a black knight, an angel or a devil, etc.?

d. With what other roles is the family having trouble?

e. If assignments are not completed, confront them about whether they really want to change and educate about family dynamics and natural resistance to changing homeostasis; challenge their ability to do so.

f. If completed, have them work one more week on the same behaviors agreed to the week before and advise them that the next week:

(1) Family therapy really begins and they are to think about whether they want to continue on this therapeutic level (i.e., trade-off), terminate, seek more intensive help, or continue with you on a more intensive level in conjunction with what they've already accomplished. Advise them that it may be threatening to return but encourage them to do so. Make positive comments about progress already made and how the family can be even further enhanced if they want to continue working with you. Offer them a chance to see another professional if time, interest, or competence are exhausted at this point.

(2) Continue to follow family with "Family Behavioral Counseling" using behavioral contracting of those specific behaviors causing family members to continue to feel specific discomforts.

Appendix B
Guide to Dynamic Family Therapy

I. Educate the family regarding how they are a system, with each member's behavior affecting the others, and how you do not see any one of them as the patient but rather the system as the patient.

II. Tell the family your interest is focused on their roles and communication within the system; therefore, during this session and the ones to follow, you want them to communicate with each other how they think the homework assignments went and you want merely to observe how they communicate. Share these observations with them from time to time during the sessions.

III. Inform the family of observations from a particular theoretical framework.

IV. Give the family an opportunity to comment and interact with each other about your observations.

V. Intervene when you see family members doing the following (adapted from Foley & Dyer, 1974):

A. not talking to one another

B. speaking for another,

C. trying to talk through you as the facilitator,

    D. inconsistencies (verbal/nonverbal especially),

    E. playing "If it weren't for them . . . ,"

    F. playing "If it weren't for you . . . ,"

    G. procrastinating or avoiding,

    H. invoking laws, or

    I. labeling.

VI. Continue to add homework assignments, now aimed at changing communication or roles within the system.

    A. Have Mom and Dad switch roles (e.g., Mom does one task Dad usually does and Dad does one task Mom does); same for the children.

    B. If using a Transactional Analysis approach, you can have the family keep a record of the times they are parented, or whatever.

VII. Later, you may want to have a longer session to continue these techniques or use more advanced techniques (e.g., family sculpture), but the family would have to be apprised that this will take longer and that they will be charged accordingly. Again, the option for referral should be raised.

References

Aluise, J. J. Human relations training for family practice residents: A four-year retrospective review. *Journal of Family Practice,* 1977, 4, 881.

Authier, J. L. The family life cycle seminar: An innovative health care psychology program. *Journal of Professional Psychology,* 1979, 10, 451-457.

Authier, J. L., & Gustafson, K. *Enriching intimacy–A behavioral approach.* Unpublished manuscript, University of Nebraska, 1973.

Authier, J. L., Starr, G. C., & Authier, K. *Family focused medicine.* Unpublished manuscript, 1979.

Bauman, M. H., & Grace, N. T. Family process and family practice. *Journal of Family practice,* 1977, 4, 1135.

Bursten, B. Family dynamics and illness behavior. *General Practitioner,* 50, 144.

Carmichael, L. P. Relational model, family ethics. Paper presented at the annual meeting of the Society of Teachers of Family Medicine, San Diego, California, May 6-9, 1978.

Fleck, S. Unified health services and family focused primary care. *International Journal of Psychiatry in Medicine,* 1975, 6, 505.

Foley, V. D., & Dyer, W. W. Timing in family therapy: The when, how and why of intervention. *Family Coordinator,* 1974, October.

Geyman, J. P. *The modern family doctor and changing medical practice.* New York: Appleton-Century-Crofts, 1971.

Geyman, J. P. The family as the object of care in family practice. *Journal of Family Practice,* 1977, 5, 571.

Haley, J. *Changing families: A family therapy reader.* Grune and Stratton, 1971.

Hill, R. Social stresses on the family. *Social Case Work,* 1958, 39, 139.

Ivey, A. E., & Authier, J. L. *Microcounseling: Innovations in interview training.* Chicago: Charles C Thomas, 1978.

Jaffe, D. T. The role of family therapy in treating physical illness. *Hospital and Community Psychology,* 1978, 29, 169-174.

Kelly, D. H. The philosophy of raising a family. *Journal of the Iowa Medical Society,* 1976, 66, 168.

Lewis, J. M. The family and physical illness. *Texas Medicine,* 1976, 72, 47-48.

Minuchin, S. The use of an ecological framework in the treatment of a child. In N. J. Anthony & C. Kaupernik (Eds.), *The child in his family.* New York: John Wiley, 1970.

Rogers, C. *Client-centered therapy.* Boston: Houghton Mifflin, 1951.

Satir, V. M. *Conjoint family therapy: A guide to theory and technique.* Palo Alto, CA: Science and Behavior Books, 1964.

Schmidt, D. D. The family as the unit of medical care. *Journal of Family Practice,* 1978, 7, 303.

Shoemaker, W. H., Tindall, H. L., Shubert, J. J., Hoke, H. H., & Argires, J. P. Chronic invalidism in a young woman: A study of family dynamics. *Journal of Family Practice,* 1977, 4, 155.

Stephens, G. G. The family physician and family therapy. *Journal of Family Practice,* 1974, 1, 70.

Truax, C. B., & Carkhuff, R. R. *Toward effective counseling and psychotherapy: Training and practice.* Chicago: AVC, 1967.

Whitaker, C. A. Psychotherapy with couples. *American Journal of Psychotherapy,* 1958, 12, 18-23.

Willard, W. Meeting the Challenge of Family Practice. Report of an Ad Hoc Committee on Education for Family Practice, Council on Medical Education. Chicago: AMA, 1966.

Young, P. Family practice in the United States.In R. B. Taylor et al. (Eds.), *Family medicine: Principles and practice.* New York: Springer-Verlag, 1978.

12

Training for Health Systems Research and Consultation

George C. Stone
University of California, San Francisco

Most of the contributions to this volume are concerned in one way or another with mental health professionals as direct providers of service to persons who have presented themselves in the health care system as recipients of service. This chapter describes an education program oriented toward a part of the health system beyond the confines of direct service. Elsewhere I have outlined the dimensions of the health system (Stone, 1979), within which the health *care* system is only a part. For example, research conducted in a department of chemistry may identify the source of a toxic substance in the atmosphere. Consumer groups may press for legislation to control the emission of the substance. Legislative bodies may commission further studies and pass laws that establish control agencies. The agencies may negotiate with industrial firms that are responsible for the pollutant to set acceptable levels of emission. According to our view of the health system, all of these interactions are *health transactions,* because health values enter into the decisions at every stage. A psychologist who studies these transactions with a view to enhancing the health outcomes that follow from them is a health psychologist.

Under this broad definition of the health system, it is at least plausible to suppose that the theories and skills in any field of psychology can be relevant to understanding and influencing the observed values of such health measures. Thus, a person becomes a health psychologist by applying whatever psychological theory and skills he or she has mastered to problems of the health system and by pursuing further expansion of those theories and skills within the settings of the health system. The task of becoming a health psychologist involves primarily the mapping of the phenomena of the health system to the abstract principles of some field of specialization in psychology.

When to Introduce Training
in Health Psychology

From this definition of the task of training health psychologists, it can be seen that there are three orders in which the two bodies of knowledge—concerning psychology and the health system—can be mastered: (1) Psychology can be learned as an academic discipline using laboratory problems and subjects as content, after which postdoctoral training, either formal or informal, provides knowledge of the health system. This is clearly the method by which most present-day health psychologists have been trained. (2) A person trained and perhaps experienced in the health system can subsequently study psychology. Quite a few present-day psychologists were originally trained as nurses. Others were first physicians, dentists, or pharmacists. (3) Knowledge of the health system can be gained *concurrently* with the study of psychology. This is the pattern provided by new, degree-oriented educational programs that offer specialization in health psychology.

We do not know at this time whether there will be systematic differences among persons who receive these different kinds of training. It seems likely that there would be differences in the professional identities that result—the physician who is also a psychologist will have passed through all those processes of socialization that impinge on medical students (Fox, 1979). Presumably, there are similar processes for students who go through the processes of graduate education in psychology, although these are surely less uniform than those that characterize education in the professions and have been studied very little (Lipsey, 1978). There may also be effects of the schemata for the organization of knowledge in the long-term memory that are operative at the time new knowledge is acquired. Is the psychology learned by someone who has already had medical training different from that of someone with an undergraduate major in psychology? Does a psychological education affect the assimilation of knowledge about the health system? Surely it must, but we can't say how. Finally, we must recognize that students who spend five years learning about both psychology and the health system in the course of acquiring a Ph.D. in health psychology may learn less about psychology than students who have the same time to spend in the study of psychology per se.

I say they may learn less, but it is not necessarily so. Inevitably, when we study any psychological *process* we must study it as it operates on some real-world content. Frequently, the content that is used to activate the processes is chosen for convenience and because we think we can control, in laboratory tasks, confounding variables. Thus, for generations associative learning was studied using nonsense syllables and contextless lists of words as the material to be learned. There has been a substantial shift recently toward the use of more meaningful materials and for studying cognitive processes in real situations, such as learning to read or solving physics problems (Larkin, McDermott, Simon, & Simon, 1980). Conceivably, students might save as much in the costs of learning about psychological processes by studying a more or less coherent set of real-world situations as they spend in learning about those situations.

What is the Domain of Health Psychology?

In the absence of empirical information, no effort will be made here to discuss the relative merits of these different approaches to the sequencing of training in health psychology. My purpose here is to consider doctoral-level programs in health psychology that provide concurrent training in psychology and the health system. More specifically, I will consider those programs that prepare their graduates to describe and analyze the processes of the health system, to identify problems that might yield to psychological interventions, and to design, test, and evaluate such interventions. In pointing to this range of activities from basic research to the delivery and evaluation of interventions, I hope to keep a broad perspective on the health system. As suggested earlier, our interest should encompass social and individual actions directed to the elimination of health hazards from the environment, the reduction of our contact with those that persist, the evaluation of information leading to the decision to seek care, and the processes of care and rehabilitation. We should be concerned not only with performing or studying the direct interventions to these ends but also with the processes by which social decisions are made, resources marshalled, programs planned and implemented, and evaluations of those programs carried out. With such a broad perspective, it becomes clear that physiological psychologists and specialists in learning, attitudes, organizations, children, families, and the aging all have a role to play.

Where to Locate Doctoral Programs in Health Psychology

I have already said that almost any type of psychological training can be relevant to health psychology. From one point of view, therefore, the broadest opportunity for acquiring psychological training would be in a large department of psychology with a full range of offerings. However, unless there are faculty members in such a department who are actively involved as health psychologists, no effective training of health psychologists can occur. Advantage can be taken of the large department to the extent that the health psychologists on the faculty have the respect and acceptance of other members of the department. The department will have to provide time in the curriculum for students to take appropriate courses in the health area. In a large department students will take their basic courses in social psychology, learning, motivation, and the like with students from all other specializations who require the same grounding in the core of the discipline. Substantive content drawn from the health system will be mixed, currently in a very small proportion, with content from many other areas. Thus, the courses will be more comprehensive and representative of the field as a whole and less focused on examples and applications in the health system. Students specializing in health psychology will be left more on their own to draw these connections.

In the past, and in the case of some fields of specialization such as educational psychology, there have been tendencies, especially in large university departments, for the more applied fields to be pushed to the periphery and for the best students to be counseled into the more abstract theory and more purified laboratory situations. These tendencies constitute hazards which may or may not have been reduced by recent social trends in relation to application of knowledge. The health system has some unique characteristics that can be used to strengthen the bonds of health psychologists to their colleagues, which I will discuss presently.

At the other pole from the large psychology department is a small group of psychologists completely committed to research and teaching in health psychology, such as the one of which I am a member at the University of California, San Francisco. The defining characteristic of this polar type of program is that the entire degree program is designed and managed by health psychologists. Core courses can be centered on health content to the degree that seems appropriate to the health psychology faculty (and to the extent that materials are available). The risk of losing touch with the main body of the discipline may be even greater here than in the case of the large department. Strong determination to remain in active contact with scientific colleagues throughout the nation is essential if this risk is to be surmounted, but more than that is required. Significant contributions to the core problems of the various fields of psychology from health psychologists working in such outposts are necessary if they are to retain full credibility and respect as psychologists.

Fortunately, several aspects of the health care system provide opportunities for health psychologists to make important contributions to psychological theory. First, the stresses people face and the decisions they are called upon to make in relation to their health problems are of the greatest consequence. Studies of the ways in which people cope with these stresses and reach these decisions can be enormously valuable in validating and extending our theories of coping and decision-making. Also, people are called upon to learn new information under a wide variety of naturally occurring states of arousal and following administration of many different kinds of drugs. Later testing for the retention of this information is entirely appropriate, in order to ensure that the patient can follow the recommended therapeutic procedures. As these examples suggest, the health system is rich with material for study.

The need for understanding the psychological aspects of these health transactions in order to enhance health outcomes for patients and health care providers alike is gaining recognition, which will increase the cooperation of potential subjects as collaborators in research. Out of subjects' understanding of the intent of the researchers to solve real and pressing problems, many ethical difficulties can be avoided that arise when the interests of researcher and subject are not so clearly associated. For example, it is difficult, if not impossible, to create significant stress or conflict in the laboratory without deceiving subjects. Also, this sense of collaboration between subject and scientist makes it possible to take advantage of generally lowered privacy barriers that prevail in health care settings to gain information that would be considered much too personal to ask about or observe in most circumstances. A final advantage to be mentioned, which facilitates the study of interventions, is the coherent value system that prevails in the health system. Unlike the worlds of business, industry, politics, and even education, where the outcomes that please some persons may displease others, in the health system all parties to the transactions that take place almost always value the health outcomes in much the same way. Of course, there remain differences of value orientation with regard to interpersonal and economic aspects of health transactions.

Training in Health Psychology at the University of California, San Francisco

Program Definition and Objectives

In the rest of this chapter I will describe a specific program in health psychology that is training psychologists for the roles of researchers, teachers, and system-level consultants in the health system. As has been said, almost any aspect of psychology could be the basis for such training. Choice of the particular set of psychological capabilities that characterize our program at UCSF was guided by a plan to enter a part of the space of possibilities that was largely devoid of training programs while it offered a promising beginning in research activity.

We began the program with a core faculty of four persons responsible for planning the curriculum and teaching most of the required courses. Their areas of specialization were cognitive, social, personality, and organizational psychology. To provide breadth in elective courses and a wealth of opportunities for supervised research, we have had a part-time faculty of about 50 persons, mostly psychologists in various programs of research and service delivery in the vast complex of hospitals and clinics associated with UCSF.

To increase the amount of teaching that could be realized from our faculty, and to create student cohorts of a size that would provide an adequate basis for student interaction and mutual support in learning activities, we designed the program to operate on a two-year cycle. Students are admitted in alternate, odd-numbered years, and the list of courses offered is markedly different in first and second years of the cycle.

The program was designed to focus on the questions of how the stresses of peoples' lives and their manner of coping with these stresses impinge on their health, how they behave in order to maintain and restore their health, and how they make their decisions about the kinds of health care services they will use. Because our program is located within a school of medicine, we have elected to concentrate on the health services of the health care system, although we emphasize to our students the importance of services and activities that go on outside of that system in such areas as health education, health economics, and health legislation.

We have conceived the future roles of our graduates to be those of collaborators with the various professions that plan, administer, and staff health care organizations. Our graduates are not to be providers of service to patients; they are not to be traditional academics who may come to observe and return to describe in the journals of their disciplines how the health system operates. We train them to be active participants in the system, choosing their research questions from among those whose answers can make an immediate difference in patterns of health care. We encourage them to join with physicians, nurses, or dentists as coinvestigators. However, our training differs from many kinds of applied programs in its deemphasis of purely empirical and pragmatic approaches and its strong emphasis on drawing from and contributing to psychological theory. We seek to apply our theories to the design, operation, and appraisal of health care organizations and to revise them on the basis of the results obtained.

The previous paragraphs outline our program objectives with regard to content. We evaluate the success of our program in conventional ways—by looking at the places where our students find employment, their success in getting their research funded, and the number and quality of their publications. Our evaluations also include a less traditional area: We are beginning to ask whether the operation of the program permits those who are involved in it to live in ways that correspond to emerging precepts about psychological aspects of health. We consider the quality of the interpersonal relationships in the program, the levels of satisfaction and self-esteem that are engendered, as well as the levels of stress that develop. We have by no means found a way to incorporate all that we think necessary in doctoral education while keeping working hours short and stress-free and eliminating frustration, failure, and conflict from the scene. In fact, we do not think that is the problem to be solved. Our achievement in this area to date is simply the admission of such considerations as legitimate governing variables (Argyris & Schön, 1974) to be monitored as the program evolves.

Historical Considerations

The program described above was grafted to an existing research training program. The earlier program, begun in 1966, had been using an apprentice model augmented by some breadth requirements. It was designed to take students from the master's level of training in psychology, or a closely related field, to the doctorate level by an extended period of work in one of the many specialized research groups of the UCSF extended campus. Twenty-four students have received Ph.D.s from this program, and 11 remain in that program at this time. Areas of specialization in this initial program, determined by the research of the participating faculty, were concentrated in biological psychology and personality psychology.

As planning for the new broadened specialization that we were calling "health psychology" got under way in 1975, the personality area of the earlier program was incorporated into it. The remaining, biological psychology component of the program continued to operate as it had before, with highly individualized curricula tailored to the specific interests of each student/faculty combination, until 1980. Experience with the first two cohorts of health psychology students, who matriculated in 1977 and 1979, led to a decision to bring the biopsychology portion of our program under the rubric of health psychology, and to have the students in that program go through a core of training that would overlap substantially with that which we had been giving to students in the social/personality/organizational (SPO) component of the program. This decision was influenced by our emerging recognition of the kinds of learning that were important for those who were preparing for careers of research, teaching, and consultation in the health care system, and by our perception that most of our students in biopsychology were, in fact, headed for such careers.

Designing the Curriculum

The program definition required that our students be strongly linked to the central core of psychology, very thoroughly grounded in research methods, and prepared to work with the people and settings of the health care system. Figure 12.1 shows the curriculum as it was defined for the third cohort of students, who matriculated in 1981. Required courses are heavily concentrated in the first two years, especially in the first year, both to provide preparation for later work and because we have found it hard to hold more advanced students to the relatively rigid formats of these courses.

The basic psychology courses of the first year are taught much as they might be taught in any academic program, although they make more use of materials from the literature of health psychology than would usually be the case. However, there is not yet much material available that links health problems to the central theoretical issues of psychology. In the social psychology course, as last taught, students read papers on "Somato-psychics and attribution" (Rodin, 1978), on parents' reactions to the sex of their child (Rothbart & Maccoby, 1966), and on applications of social-psychological theory to the health field (Janis & Rodin, 1979; Taylor, 1978). The rest of their readings were drawn from conventional sources. The course on personality assigned two readings related to health out of a total of 29, one on "Psychological traits and serum lipids" (Jenkins, Hames, Zyzanski, Rosenman, & Friedman, 1969) and one on "Stressful life events, personality and

---

FIGURE 12.1: Curriculum Description for Third Cohort

Curriculum

Students granted a Ph.D. in this program will be trained in research methods, statistics, basic theories of psychology, and in one of two specialty areas: Social-Personality-Organizational or Biobehavioral. They will also have the opportunity to take electives, a partial list of which is given below. The goal of the program is to produce psychologists who have well-developed research skills, an understanding of the health care system, and a mastery of conceptual frameworks in which problems of health and illness can be examined.

(Continued)

Requirements For Ph.D.

Social-Personality-Organizational Division	Biobehavioral Division
	2 of the following 3:
Learning & Cognition	Learning & Cognition
Personality Psychology	Personal Psychology
Social Psychology	Social Psychology
Statistics A, B, & C	Statistics A, B, & C
Personality-Social-Organizational Research Methods	Bio-behavioral Research Methods
Introduction to Health Psychology	Introduction to Health Psychology
Physiological Aspects of Health Psychology	Human Physiological Psychology
Health Research Colloquium A, B, & C (1 unit each)	Health Research Colloquium A, B, & C (1 unit each)
Research Placement and Seminar A, B, & C	Research Placement and Seminar A, B, & C
The Health System	One course outside Department (e.g., Neuroanatomy, Biochemistry, Pharmacology)
	3rd year Proseminar
5 elective courses	5 elective courses
Qualifying Examination	Qualifying Examination
Dissertation proposal	Dissertation proposal
Dissertation	Dissertation

Electives (partial listing):

Psychophysiology of Consciousness
Impact of Health Insurance and Legislation on Practice
Communication Skills
Program Evaluation in Health and Human Service Organizations
Psychological Stress and Coping
Stress and Bodily Disease
Health Transactions
Individual and Society: Psychoanalysis and Social Science
Reproductive Behavior
Clinical Approaches to Psychological Disorders
Introduction to the Computer for Behavioral Sciences
Tests and Measurement
Hemispheric Specialization and Integration
Electrophysiology

Individual tutorials, guided readings, and electives in other departments as well as at other University of California campuses may be arranged.

All courses listed earlier as required for one Division may be taken as an elective for the other.

FIGURE 12.1

health" (Kobasa, 1979). In the learning/cognition course, assignment of Miller's (1978) article on "Biofeedback and visceral learning" provided the only input of material directly related to the health care system.

Students in both program divisions take a survey course in health psychology that attempts to provide an overview of the field and the work currently being done in it. Although we maintain the viewpoint that it is important to consider all of the potential contributions of psychology, in this course we stress those areas in which substantial bodies of research are accumulating. Stress, coping, and illness; preventive health behavior; modification of self-destructive behavior; biofeedback in the treatment of illness; decision-making by clients and providers; adherence to medical regimens; and evaluation of outcomes of health care transactions are some of the topics covered. Most of these topics are, of course, considered in more detail in later courses.

The courses intended to prepare the students for working in the health care system are stressed more heavily for the students in the SPO area, since we expect that they will all be doing their research in field settings, while the students in the biobehavioral (BB) emphasis area may be spending much of their time in research laboratories. The SPO students are required to take an introductory course in human physiology and pathophysiology, so that when they interact with health professionals and health professional students they will not be ignorant of the fundamental terms and processes that are taken for granted by these people.

A ten-week course in physiology can hardly provide more than a recognition memory for the outlines of the organ systems, the most salient biochemical processes, and the descriptions of major disease entities and their treatment in these terms. Our first two cohorts of students took this course during their first quarter in the program, where it was a heavy burden during a difficult period of adaptation. Reluctantly, we have moved it to the second year, at which time we hope that the students will have a clearer recognition of the importance of this preparation. Our concern is that they should not, as a result of this delay, experience and give the impression of egregious ignorance in the health care environment. We expect that as students begin to be involved in research in a particular health care setting they will gain a deeper knowledge of the physiological and biochemical aspects of the health problems that are confronted there. Some students elect to take more advanced courses in other departments, but most find that they can read the more general parts of the medical literature with understanding as a result of this single course.

Students in the SPO division also take a course that describes the health system in the large and kinds of analyses of it made by other social and behavioral sciences. This course provides a context within which students can locate the particular problems they choose to work on. We intend it to facilitate appropriate generalization and discrimination of principles, and to develop the concept of mapping particulars to abstract frameworks. It also lays a groundwork for interdisciplinary collaboration by demonstrating alternative descriptions and analyses of the same reality. Programs in medical anthropology, medical sociology, health policy, and bioethics on our campus provide the opportunity for study of these subjects in greater depth.

Students in the BB division are encouraged to take these basic courses, but they are expected to become actively involved in research during their first year in one of the laboratories of the psychology faculty. Students in the SPO division, in contrast, are encouraged to wait until their second year before undertaking a "research placement" in a field setting. Students are guided to placements where they can be supervised by some member of the extended faculty who has already established entry and worked out a basis for gathering data. It has been our experience that most second-year students do not yet have the skills and knowledge necessary to establish a base of operation for themselves. We want the students in the second year to complete a project successfully within the nine-month period available to them, and they cannot do this if they make a false start. A product of publishable quality is one goal for these second-year projects. A year-long seminar meets in conjunction with these projects, where students discuss the issues with which they are grappling. We hope in this way to provide vicarious experience that is much broader than that an individual student confronts.

By the third year, most students are involved in one or more research projects, often as part-time employees or paid consultants. Skills of data processing, interviewing, instrument design, evaluation research, and the like are sufficiently in demand so that students who want to can work on projects that broaden their experience and lead them into new conceptual areas.

The curriculum from the third year on is highly individualized. Students first identify a set of three or four topic areas for intensive preparation, and then immerse themselves in the literature of those areas in preparation for written and oral qualifying examinations, taken near the end of the third or the beginning of the fourth year in the program. Students are guided in their definitions of the topic areas to span the range from the theoretical core of psychology to specific applications to health issues. Below are examples of recent topic sets.

I. The social nature of psychological research.
  The social psychology of organizational leadership.
  Evaluation research in the health field.

II. Theories of behavior change.
Psychological factors in the development of bodily illness.
Understanding risk factor behavior.

By the end of the second year students can largely assume responsibility for their own educations. The major challenges of the qualifying exams and the dissertation are there to be met, but the means for doing so are left to the students. Faculty are available for support, counsel, and facilitation of access to needed resources. We gauge the success of this reliance on student initiative by accomplishments of the students on their way to mastery of the subject matter. Examples of the kinds of opportunities that our first cohort have found for themselves include the experiences of two students who have spent one or two summers working for the World Health Organization in Geneva on research projects concerned with the acceptability of various means for male and female contraception. Another student organized a research team of faculty and medical experts and wrote a response to a "Request for Proposal" from the National Heart, Lung and Blood Institute that brought to UCSF a three-year, $490,000 contract. The student was named project director and will do her dissertation research as an augmentation of one of the phases of the project. Preparation of the proposal and preparation for the qualifying examination were done simultaneously and led to a mastery of the literature in the areas of evaluation of educational systems and the dissemination and utilization of knowledge that was the basis for excellent performance in both tasks.

Our program objectives include preparing our students for teaching roles, both with students of psychology and with health professional students. This preparation is an aspect of our program that has posed special difficulties because of our location on a campus with no undergraduate students. We are able to make a few teaching opportunities available to advanced students in courses offered to our beginning students. We have also begun to involve our students in electives offered to health professional students. This avenue is limited at present by the degree of recognition by health professionals of the relevance of psychological material to their practice and by intense competition among all the departments of the campus for the scarce elective time of health professional students. We anticipate a gradual increase in acceptance as our presence as research collaborators expands.

Recruitment, Selection, and Retention of Students

Recruitment for each of our first two cohorts of students, in 1977 and 1979, made use of a single announcement published in the *APA Monitor,* the monthly newspaper of the American Psychological Association, and a one-page flyer mailed to psychology departments in most colleges and universities in the United States. These very modest recruitment efforts, which stressed the nonclinical, research-oriented training we were offering, brought us about 100 applicants in 1977 and nearly as many in 1979, from whom we selected 10 and 14 to receive offers of admission. We were unable to promise financial support to any students, although one or two in each cohort won a regent's fellowship in competition with applicants to all graduate programs on our campus.

In addition to the usual criteria of prior academic records and performance on the Graduate Record Examination, we looked for indications of a mature commitment to research in the health system. Previous research experience was the strongest indicator, followed by either paid or volunteer experience working in a health setting which had given rise to thoughtful questions about the operation of the system. We did not choose applicants whose stated goals or interest patterns revealed that they were drawn to clinical work. The success of this screening may be judged by the fact that only one of our original cohort has since shifted to a clinical program and one other (chosen for other reasons in spite of an absence of experience with the health system) has left for training in an area outside of psychology. The others remain committed to careers in research, teaching, and consultation, as we had hoped they would.

The groups we selected were approximately balanced between males and females, but we were able to attract only one qualified applicant from an ethnic minority group, and have lost him. Although we had originally designed the program to build upon the bachelor's degree in psychology, we have admitted only six students who did not have master's degrees. Our emphasis on experience in the selection criteria gives an advantage to somewhat older, more mature students. The median age of our first cohort was 27; of our second, 25.

When we chose our first cohort of students in February 1977, health psychology was an almost unknown field and our program was totally untested. Our offers were accepted by only six of the first 10 to whom they were extended. Several students with high academic qualifications accepted offers from other schools that were better known and had more financial aid to offer. Our second cohort of applicants, in 1979, presented a somewhat higher set of GRE scores. The average values for students offered positions in the program was 1280, in contrast to an average of 1175 for our first offers. We made 14 initial offers to this second group, in order to fill our allotment of 10 students. To our surprise, 12 accepted.

Evaluation of the Program

We are very pleased with the results from our program to date, but we recognize that they are very preliminary, since no student has yet graduated from the health psychology program. We appear to be accomplishing at least two of the three major program objectives stated earlier. Students entering their fourth year in the program are very competent in research methods, including the design and analysis of data from field studies and quasi-experiments. They are already able to perform on a par with professionals in the field. They have learned enough about the health care system to be able to function in it as full-fledged members of that system. Their professional identities as competent researchers provide them with the basis for collaborating effectively with research-oriented providers of health services. Evidence with regard to our third major objective, development of a pattern of drawing from and contributing to the core knowledge and theory of psychology, is not yet available.

Plans for our future include the development of a colloquium series that will not only bring outstanding health psychologists to our campus but will also invite theoreticians who have not been identified with the health system as a substantive context to consider the applicability of their theories to the phenomena that we observe.

There is no doubt in our minds that health psychology has become a fully viable field in psychology. We anticipate that it will continue to flourish both as a clinical branch of the profession of psychology and as an area of specialization for basic and applied research.

References

Argyris, C., & Schön, D. A. *Theory in practice: Increasing professional effectiveness.* San Francisco: Jossey-Bass, 1974.

Fox, R. C. Is there a "new" medical student? A comparative view of medical socialization in the 1950's and the 1970's. In R. C. Fox et al. (Eds.), *Essays in medical sociology.* New York: John Wiley, 1979.

Janis, I. L., & Rodin, J. Attribution, control and decision making: Social psychology and health care. In G. C. Stone, F. Cohen, & N. E. Adler (Eds.), *Health psychology: A handbook.* San Francisco: Jossey-Bass, 1979.

Jenkins, C. D., Hames, C. G., Zyzanski, S. J., Rosenman, R. H., & Friedman, M. Psychological traits and serum lipids. *Psychosomatic Medicine,* 1969, 31, 115-128.

Kobasa, S. C. Stressful life events, personality and health: An inquiry into hardiness. *Journal of Personality and Social Psychology,* 1979, 37, 1-11.

Larkin, J., McDermott, J., Simon, D. P., & Simon, H. A. Expert and novice performance in solving physics problems. *Science,* 1980, 208, 1335-1342.

Lipsey, M. W. Occupational socialization and mid-career orthodoxy among academic psychologists. *Personality and Social Psychology Bulletin,* 1978, 4, 169-172.

Miller, N. E. Biofeedback and visceral learning. *Annual Review of Psychology,* 1978, 29, 373-404.

Rodin, J. Somatopsychics and attribution. *Personality and Social Psychology Bulletin,* 1978, 4, 531-540.

Rothbart, M. K., & Maccoby, E. E. Parents' differential reactions to sons and daughters. *Journal of Personality and Social Psychology,* 1966, 4, 1-7.

Stone, G. C. Health and the health system: A historical overview and conceptual framework. In G. C. Stone, F. Cohen, & N. E. Adler (Eds.), *Health psychology: A handbook.* San Francisco: Jossey-Bass, 1979.

Taylor, S. A developing role for social psychology in medicine and medical practice. *Personality and Social Psychology Bulletin,* 1978, 4, 515-523.

PART IV

RESEARCH AND EVALUATION OF COORDINATED CARE

13

Evaluating Integrated Service Delivery Systems

C. Clifford Attkisson
University of California, San Francisco
Anthony Broskowski
Northside Community Mental Health Center, Inc.
Tampa, Florida

Introduction

Significant service integration research issues can be identified across a wide range of evaluation targets and organizational levels of the health and human services system. This chapter attempts to summarize the research issues at the levels of clinical epidemiology, service utilization, clinical practice, organizational arrangements, and the role of government in service delivery and funding.

Clinical Epidemiology

Some of the important research questions in this area are as follows:

- In any one year, how many new (incidence) and existing (prevalence) cases of diagnosed emotional disorders are there?

- How are these cases distributed geographically and across sociodemographic strata?

- What is the relative frequency of specific types of disorders?

- How many of these cases of emotional disorders have concurrent medical problems? Are there any significant cause-effect relationships between medical and psychological problems, or are they independent?

Answering these questions requires development and refinement of reliable and valid diagnostic instruments, appropriate sampling methods, multisite collaboration, and the continuity of funding to support longitudinal studies.

Clinical Practice and Service Utilization

Information about the incidence and prevalence of emotional disorders must be coupled with an understanding of service utilization patterns and the methods of professional practice used by service providers.

- How many persons with a diagnosed disorder use a health and/or mental health service?

- Do persons with emotional disorders use more health services than those without such disorders? Is this use appropriate?

- Do persons with emotional disorders receiving mental health care use less primary health care services? How do primary health care needs among these persons change over time?

- What are the effects of different behavioral lifestyles on rates of morbidity and mortality?

- What is the level of untreated prevalence for a given time period?

- What is the capacity of the specialty sector and the primary health care sector to treat the known prevalence of emotional disorders?

- What are the methods for detection, diagnosis, and treatment, and do these methods differ when we compare specialty mental health care providers and primary health care providers?

- Does increasing the mental health knowledge of primary care providers change their ability to detect and diagnose, or their methods of treatment?

- Are different methods of treatment (within the primary care sector) associated with differences in patient outcomes?

In addition to problems associated with instrumentation, sampling, collaboration, and funding, answers to these questions depend upon the quality of information and record systems within service institutions. Without adequate records documenting patient problems and care provided, these questions cannot be answered. Definitive answers will require evaluative research designs using control groups and planned interventions.

Organizational Arrangements

Research questions in this area are concerned with the effects of different patterns of organizing, linking, and financing services. Obtaining answers to these questions is contingent upon the adequacy of research in the areas of clinical epidemiology and service utilization.

- What is the effect of liaison staff on the continuity of care across multiple organizations?

- What are the administrative and financial barriers to interagency cooperation?

- How do service reimbursement systems provide incentives for prevention, early treatment, and health maintenance?

- Within primary care settings, are there cost savings when mental health components are included in the range or organizational services?

- How much of the observed reduction in primary health care utilizations after mental health utilization is due to

  a. the type and amount of mental health services received,

  b. the effect of the services on the physical condition,

  c. the effect of the service on the psychological condition,

  d. the client, still in need of health care, leaving the system prematurely and inappropriately, or

  e. the effect of the service on improving the patient's compliance with the treatment of the physical problem?

Research on organizational arrangements requires the cooperation of service organizations whose primary mission is service and not research. The research methodologies most applicable are systems or operations research, econometrics, and large-scale controlled demonstrations that manipulate organizational variables. The cooperation and methodologies necessary for this area of research require long-range planning, large-scale financial commitment, and adequate answers to the research questions in areas of clinical epidemiology and clinical practice.

Governmental Sponsorship

Research questions in this area focus on the impact of federal, state, and local government resources, policies, and procedures on the integration of health and mental health services. The important issues include the role of government as the owner and operator of services, equity in the distribution of available resources, and the differential impact of alternative funding and regulatory mechanisms.

- What is the impact of restrictive eligibility requirements on accessibility and continuity of care?

- Will block grant funding of health and human services have any impact on availability, accessibility, continuity, and cost of services?

- Will curtailment of regulations result in cost savings, service efficiency, and continuity without corresponding reductions in the equity of service distribution and quality?

- What are the relative advantages and disadvantages of government purchasing services rather than operating service agencies directly?

The research methods used here are a blend of policy research and analysis, case studies, and controlled comparisons of alternative policies and procedures. The clarity and validity of such analysis will, of course, depend on the grace of God (Rabkin & Silverman, 1979).

The Context of Integration Research

We have identified key research questions in four major areas. These research issues are embedded within a broader context of evaluation targets, sponsors, objectives, and methodologies. The targets and sponsors of integration research span the breadth of the health and human service (HHS) system ranging from the level of the individual citizen to the national government.

The HHS system, as a conceptual entity, has vertical dimensions progressing from service delivery to a complex array of planning, administrative, and regulatory structures. Along this vertical dimension resources are brokered and allocated according to a mix of force fields, including those of equity, privilege, ideology, and social power. These are the force fields that have produced such phenomena as the "categorical" program apparatus, revenue sharing, PSRO, and health systems agencies, to mention only a few. At every level of the vertical dimension there are lateral or horizontal interconnections that are far less robust and less influential than the vertical structures. The lateral plane exists only conceptually at most levels, without the formalized linkages that characterize the vertical plane. Attempts to strengthen lateral structures are invariably faced with resistance from the vested vertical interests: categorical ideology, strains toward equity, counterpressures from privileged groups, the brokers of social power in legislatures, specialized bureaucracies, professional associations, and specific population groups. Such forces constrain efforts to integrate HHS programs at all levels from the community to the President's Cabinet. Perhaps the greatest source of resistance is the threat that categorical interests will lose their clear identity or specificity of purpose. It is more difficult to manage a program that is too generalized, too fragmented by external commitments, and too removed from a clear-cut claim of support from specific and well-defined political alliances.

Evaluation of horizontal integrative linkages must take into account the vertical force fields that resist or facilitate such linkages. In short, integrative efforts must cope with vertical force fields and must be shaped to adjust for resistance based on perceived threats to vertical identity and to the strains of fragmentation.

Integrative structures can be designed within every horizontal level of the HHS system, although the integrative goals, objectives, and strategies may differ significantly from level to level as they apply to each successive configuration. Similarly, at each horizontal level *evaluation* efforts will have differing targets, sponsors, objectives, and methodologies. This array is portrayed in Table 13.1.

At each vertical level, defined in Table 13.1 by the *target* of the evaluation, there are multiple potential sponsors. Sponsors at higher levels are usually represented at all lower levels. Therefore, lower levels simultaneously endure multiple evaluation strategies imposed upon them independently by several higher levels. Typically, very little horizontal colloboration occurs at higher levels in planning those evaluation efforts that focus on lower levels.

Integrative methods lead to specific evaluation strategies that evolve from more generic evaluative methodologies. Table 13.1 addressed these evaluative methodologies by reviewing, for each HHS system level,

- the target level of the evaluation,
- the sponsors of the evaluation,
- the purposes of the evaluation.

TABLE 13.1 Targets, Sponsors, Objectives, and Methods in Evaluating Integrated Delivery Systems

TARGETS (What is evaluated)	SPONSORS (Who does the evaluation)	OBJECTIVES (Purposes of the evaluation)	METHODS (How it is done)
Client Level: Individuals or Groups of Clients	• Service Agency, Administrative and Clinical Staff • Governmental Funding or Regulatory Agency • Commercial or Academic Research Organization • External Peer Review Agency • Consumer or Advocacy Groups	• To enhance clinical, administrative decisions • To improve patient compliance, satisfaction, and outcomes • To assess level and distribution of needs • To produce new knowledge	• Measuring patient's functional status • Quality assurance • Patient self-evaluation • Goal attainment scaling • Monitoring service use • Clinical trials • Comparative studies of utilization and outcomes • Epidemiological surveys
Service Provider Level: Clinicians or Groups of Clinicians	• Service Agency • Accreditation Agency • Professional Associations • Governmental Funding or Regulatory Agency • Commercial or Academic Research Organization • Consumer or Advocacy Groups	• To evaluate productivity • To assess provider competency • To assure compliance with professional standards • To assess personnel availability and distribution • To assess future training and personnel needs • To evaluate outcomes by types of providers	• Production by studies • Accreditation and licensing visits measuring compliance with measurable standards • Assessment of professional knowledge • Measuring effects of continuing education • Controlled studies of efforts to change provider's knowledge, skills, or attitudes

TABLE 13.1 Continued

Service Delivery Level	Purposes	Methods
Single or Multipurpose Service Agencies • Service Agency • Board of Directors • Governmental Funding, Regulatory, or Planning Agencies • Legislative Bodies • Judicial Entities • Commercial or Academic Research Organization • Accreditation Agencies	• To evaluate agency productivity and service quality • To assess compliance with standards • To plan new services • To improve efficiency or reduce costs	• Management information systems to assess level of effort, outcome, adequacy, and efficiency • Cost and resource accounting • Site visits to assess records for indicators of measurable goals and objectives • Special studies of patient outcomes, continuity, and referral patterns • Patient satisfaction studies • Special surveys and research projects to assess interagency linkages
Substate Level: Private or Government Agencies or Constellations of Service Organizations • Local Government Agency • Regional or District Level of State Agency • Health Systems Agency • Consumer/Advocacy Group • Consortium of Service Provider Agencies • Research Organizations	• To assess current levels of service integration • To guide comprehensive service planning • To assess equity of resource allocations • To assess needs for future linkages	• Assess accomplishment of planned objectives • Assess barriers to linkage • Monitor use of specialized linkage resources • Trace existing referral and utilization patterns • Measure continuity of care for target groups
State Level: Private or Government Entities or Legislative Body • State "Umbrella" Agency • State Program Agency • State Legislature	• To assess compliance with legislative intent, statutes, rules and	• Programmatic and fiscal audits, site visits, etc. • Monitoring through use

(Continued)

TABLE 13.1 Continued

• State Audit Agency • State Health Care Coordinating Council • Consumer/Advocacy/Special Interest Groups • Commercial or Academic Research Organization	regulations with respect to structural, procedural, or financial requirements • To guide future policy or legislation • To assess equity of resource allocations • To coordinate activities across the array of state-level agencies	of minimal data sets on providers, clients, and services • Policy research • Needs assessment surveys • Special studies or demonstrations and evaluation projects
National Level: Private or Government Entities • Congress and the GAO • Executive Cabinet Department • Office of Management and Budget • Other Regulation Entities (e.g., FDA) • Federal Program Agencies • National Consumer, Advocacy, or Special Interest Groups • Commercial or Academic Research Organization	• To assess compliance with Congressional intent and existing statutes, rules, and regulations • To guide future policies and legislation • To assess equity of revenue allocations • To generate new knowledge and ideas • To coordinate activities across the array of federal agencies	• Programmatic and fiscal audits, site visits, etc. • Policy and evaluation research • Special clinical research demonstrations and evaluation projects • Monitoring through use of minimal data sets and in-depth sampling • Cost-outcome-benefit analyses

This conceptual framework assumes that evaluation of service integration is embedded, inexorably, within the total HHS evaluation enterprise. Evaluation of service integration presumes a broad base of information, much of it collected for other purposes. In fact, evaluators of service integration efforts may be primarily consumers of information generated by others for a host of other evaluative, statistical, and accountability purposes. To be sure, however, evaluations of integration efforts bring a unique perspective to the analysis of available information, especially as available information is combined with new data collected specifically to address key questions about the integration of services. In addition, evaluators of integration are equally torn between lateral and hierarchical strains as they pursue their objectives. They too must compete for time and resources that are all too scarce at the lower systemic levels.

The balance of this chapter will follow Table 13.1 to discuss the integration and evaluation activities that occur at each level of the HHS system. In turn, we will identify the typical sponsors, purposes, and methodologies of evaluation at each level.

Client Level: Individuals or Groups of Clients

Sponsors at this level include individual clinicians who evaluate and diagnose patient needs at patient entry, during treatment, at exit, and possibly at multiple follow-up points. This information is used for clinical decision-making, for referral decisions based on the range of patient needs, and for formal documentation to be used by quality assurance personnel in peer review, profile analysis, utilization review, and clinical audits of various kinds. Government funding and regulatory agencies require ongoing documentation of patient characteristics, service utilization, and clinical satisfactions and outcomes. External peer review agencies use clinical record and information system documentation to ensure quality of care in agencies where quality assurance has not been delegated by the PSRO to the specific agency. Consumer or patient advocacy groups request or demand aggregate patient data to use in their reviews of clinical adequacy and responsiveness to community needs. Academic researchers or private research organizations are continuously involved in data collection at this level for purposes of assessing clinical or theoretical hypotheses. Such studies are a major source of new knowledge about the efficacy of innovations or the etiology of a disease or dysfunctional state.

Two of the most important sponsors of evaluation studies at the individual patient level are agency administrators and epidemiological researchers. Agency administrators, including executives, middle managers, and evaluators, use client-level information to support and enhance administrative decisions. The decisions range from the long-range planning of agency needs to personnel evaluations, including data on program effort and utilization, program outcomes, cost-efficiency, and service adequacy relative to the broader community needs for services.

Epidemiologists have an equally important, though relatively less frequent, need for client-level information to determine incidence and prevalence rates, service utilization patterns, and the cooccurrence of primary health care needs and emotional disorders. These data are combined for multiple sites to specify the magnitude of need for mental health services and to estimate the untreated prevalence. Epidemiological surveys require instruments having known high levels of sensitivity and specificity to mental disorder. These instruments must be used with very large representative community and institutional samples to allow for detection of rare disorders.

Typically, information about the individual level is specific to data collected from patients in treatment. The most frequently used methodologies include functional status measures, patient satisfaction and self-evaluation measures, goal attainment scaling techniques, clinical trials research strategies, and comparative studies of utilization and outcome, including profile analyses. Less typically, information about the individual level is collected in random, stratified samples of the general population.

Service Provider Level:
Clinicians or Groups of Clinicians

Service providers are *the* principal resource in the labor-intensive field of health and human services. Increasingly provider groups are being assessed as a key aspect of health economics research. Those sponsoring these evaluations include service delivery agencies which must make ongoing decisions about personnel effectiveness, comply with quality assurance structural standards, and review the adequacy of personnel relative to the changing mix of patient needs and characteristics. Beyond the level of the service agency, many other entities are very interested in information about service providers by discipline, credentials, areas of specialization, and practice patterns. These other groups include accrediting agencies, professional associations, governmental funding and regulatory agencies, research organizations, and consumer/advocacy groups.

The general purposes of evaluation of providers and provider groups include the need for data on compliance with professional standards, assessment of provider competency, assessment of personnel availability and distribution, and evaluation of productivity. In addition, information is collected about outcomes by type of provider and about future training and personnel needs.

The most frequently used methodologies are surveys, site visits, and the use of existing data bases created by professional associations or service agencies. Organizations at the national, state, and local levels are frequently assessing the knowledge or training needs of professional or paraprofessional service providers. Once implemented, training programs are evaluated in terms of changes in trainee's skills or such surrogate indicators as type of job or service setting in which the trainee works. The federal government has also funded specific training demonstration projects to increase the abilities of specialists, such as primary health care providers, to detect, diagnose, and treat patients with emotional disorders. Government agencies also monitor service provider availability and distribution through the use of surveys and reports required to be completed by government-funded or licensed service providers or service agencies.

Service Delivery Level

Sponsors at this level include the boards of directors of service agencies; governmental funding, regulatory, and planning agencies; legislative bodies; judicial entities; commercial or academic research organizations; and accreditation agencies. These sponsors typically are interested in an agency's productivity, service quality, compliance with standards or policies, and overall efficiency in the use of limited resources. Assessment of existing resources and unmet need or demand for services are used to develop plans for new services.

The methods used to carry out such assessments generally rely on the agency's management information system, coupled with other existing internal record systems and the collection of new data from inside or outside the agency (Broskowski and Attkisson, in press). Budgetary and cost data are commonly examined to determine how financial resources are being used. Accreditation agencies, such as the Joint Commission on Accreditation of Hospitals (JCAH), examine a tremendous volume of the service agency's paperwork, including medical records, administrative memos and correspondence, staff and board meeting minutes, and the documentation of efforts to conduct service evaluations and needs assessments.

Of special concern for purposes of integrated care are the special studies carried out to determine the multiple needs of clients and whether or not these needs are being met internally or through formal affiliation agreements and informal referral practices. Client satisfaction and outcome studies may also address continuity concerns. Legislative and judicial bodies have shown particular interest in the needs of the high-risk patient and the responsibility of the service agency to allocate internal resources in the most equitable manner. Despite such pressures, however, fragmentation at the higher levels of governmental organization also work against an equitable allocation at the service level. For example, the bulk of health and mental health dollars continue to be spent on hospital-based care, for acute medical conditions and chronic mental disorders.

Substate Level

Some states divide themselves into regions or districts, and some into smaller service areas. Clinical and funding authority may or may not be decentralized in such substate entities. States also vary in respect to the degree of county or municipal government participation. Of course, health systems agencies, required by PL 93-641, represent another type of substate entity. All of these entities have an interest in linkage development and evaluation. Also, at this level it is possible to see a consortium of service providers or a consumer advocacy group play a role in linkage planning and evaluation. University faculty or research contractors also operate at this level.

At the substate level it becomes possible realistically to consider studies focused on the level of service integration for the citizens/consumers living in the defined geographical area. For example, studies may examine the flow of patients among multiple service settings or the pattern of problems and services within single settings with multiple services. Many of the service integration studies, sponsored by DHEW (John, 1977), examined such relationships.

Evaluations may also take the form of examining the accomplishment of planned objectives on a community-wide basis. Are behavioral emergencies being attended by mental health professionals in general hospitals? Are liaison staff being hired to assist in case consultation and interagency referrals? Is inservice training on mental health resources being provided to local pediatricians and other primary care providers? Such goals, to the extent that they are identified, provide the basis for further study and evaluations.

Needs assessments, including an analysis of current resources and utilization patterns, are best conducted at this level (Siegel, Attkisson, & Carson, 1978). Needs assessments at this level can also examine specific barriers to integrated care, such as transportation, cultural, and social factors that are difficult to address in state-level planning.

To the extent that funding decisions are made by substate entities or local governments, evaluations of coordinated care can be linked to financial incentives. Funding priorities for the coordination of health and mental health services to particular target groups, such as children, the elderly, or the chronically mentally ill, can also be set at the substate level if budgetary discretion exists there.

Service organizations at this level may choose to plan specific linkages and conduct a self-evaluation of their effectiveness. A range of interorganizational models (see Chapter 9)—including the exchanges of clients, staff, services, or information—can be planned, implemented, and evaluated for their impact on the continuity of care, costs, and client outcomes.

State Level

There are wide variations among the 50 states in how they currently organize and integrate categorical health and mental health services. Their integration evaluation interests and capabilities will vary accordingly. In some states health and mental health are separate agencies, but each is controlled by an "umbrella"-level organization. Such umbrella agencies, however, may vary considerably in their concern that these separate agencies actually work together. For example, Hagedorn (Chapter 3) provides a brief glimpse at state-level struggles to meet the coordinated health planning requirements imposed on states by the federal government. What will happen if there is no federal requirement? With increasing flexibility and increasing responsibility to allocate federal dollars, state legislative and administrative agencies may go either way.

Another major determinant of the state's ability or interest in evaluating coordinated care will be its pattern of operating on funding services. For example, in some states many mental health centers and clinics are directly owned and operated by the state. In other states, the policy is to purchase community-based services from private nonprofit agencies. In the former states administrative control is likely to be seen as an adequate basis for monitoring and evaluation. When the state purchases care it is likely to be more motivated to monitor and evaluate. It is not uncommon to see a state exercise two levels of standards, one for state-operated clinics and another for the private sector, proprietary, or nonprofit.

The capacity to engage in evaluation activities is highly variable across states and when comparing health agencies with mental health agencies within the same state. Evaluators in separate state agencies seldom work together and are more likely to have disparate types of professional training and use different evaluation technologies. The degree to which the monitoring and evaluation functions are tied to the planning and resource allocation functions will also vary widely. In some states the legislative branch is dominant in planning through its budgetary process. In other states the administrative branches are more influential.

In the immediate future we are likely to witness confusion and chaos in most state efforts to evaluate coordinated care. The emphasis is likely to remain on fiscal audits, program audits through statistical reporting, site visits, and, in some states, statewide needs assessments.

In a few states, where separate administrative and legislative branches can successfully work together, there is a good potential for specialized research and demonstration projects. For example, Medicaid represents a significant cost item in any state's total budget of state dollars. It would be in the interest of the state legislature to consider the potential financial savings if a "cost-offset" effect could be demonstrated in settings where Medicaid utilization is high. Such a demonstration, of course, would require overcoming the established domains of separate administrative agencies and the special interests of powerful service provider groups.

A state's interests in special problems, such as services for the urban poor or deinstitutionalization, may prove to be the determining factor in its interests in and capability to evaluate coordinated care. By focusing on such special targets as the poor, the elderly, the chronically physically and mentally ill, and children, a state is in a good position to discover the potentials of coordinated care. The evaluation of state priorities in such areas could well move the art of program evaluation beyond the narrow focus on single outcomes of specialized services.

National Level

The major roles of national-level entities in the evaluation of integrated services can be arbitrarily divided between the legislative and executive branches of the federal government. Private organizations, including consumer or professional interest groups, research and consulting firms, and universities, also become involved, commonly serving under grants and contracts from the government, and sometimes independently.

The history of categorical legislation in the U.S. Congress provides a very thin and narrow foundation for evaluations of congressional intent with respect to integrated services. In fact, it has been more commonly the

Congress's intent to keep the flow of money, power, services, information, and other resources within the familiar narrow channels. The Government Accounting Office (GAO), as the evaluation agency of Congress, has shown very little interest in special studies to examine the health/mental health connection.

This condition, however, may not be perpetuated because of the inflationary crisis. For example, Congress will be considering President Reagan's proposal for block grants that combine multiple categorical programs into a single allocation to each state. Congress took a timid step toward coordinating health and mental health care in passing the Mental Health Systems Act, which includes grants to create linkages between CMHCs and ambulatory health settings (See Chapters 2 and 9). Of course, Congress has passed numerous pieces of legislation that call for "better coordination," but the actual dollars and administrative linkages to truly implement such endeavors has seldom been forthcoming. In fact, Congress has been reluctant to consider seriously efforts to promote integration when it was presented with model legislation, such as the Allied Services Act, by the Nixon administration. Congressional intent is hard to fathom, much less evaluate, because it is commonly interpreted by the staff of the administrative branch of government, who are loyal to the specialized categorical interests of their professional constituencies.

Most of the impetus and responsibility for evaluation of integrated services at the national level resides in the administrative branch. At the cabinet level, the connection between health and mental health would clearly fall within the Department of Health and Human Service (DHHS). However, barring a special interest in integrated services, such as that shown by former DHEW Secretary Eliot Richardson, the Cabinet level of government has little capacity to focus on integration or evaluation. Special sections within DHHS are charged to do special evaluation studies, but these commonly have little impact on subsequent policy-making or legislation. Most of the "action" in service planning and evaluation occurs at the subcabinet level, where service grants and contracts are distributed and monitored. Recent steps at the level of Alcohol, Drug, and Mental Health Administration (ADAMHA) and the Health Resources Administration (HRA) to promote demonstration of coordinated planning and delivery of mental health and health services suggest that the categorical boundaries at these levels are breaking down. Special demonstrations of linkages between health and mental health have been funded by the Bureau of Community Health Services (BCHS) and subsequently evaluated by the National Institute of Mental Health (NIMH). Chapter 2, by Burns, Burke, and Kesseler, and Chapter 9, by Marks and Broskowski, provide additional details to suggest the types of evaluation and research that need to be directed and funded by agencies at this level of government.

Both health and mental health agencies at the federal level may choose to use their categorically earmarked research and demonstration funds to assess the need and evaluate the benefits of noncategorical approaches. For example, the National Center for Health Services Delivery Research has stimulated research on behavioral emergencies in hospital emergency rooms (See Chapter 15 by Elinor Walker), and NIMH has funded studies on the magnitude of the cost-offset effect (See Chapter 14 by Mumford, Schleslinger, and Glass).

Efforts to cut federal spending may have opposing effects on the evaluation of coordinated care. In one respect, such strategies as block grants may allow greater flexibility at the state level to initiate such activities (assuming the leadership and creativity exist at that level). On the other hand, federal reductions in spending for coordinated health planning and cost-containment, to reduce the regulatory pressures on hospitals, will further diminish the power of integrative planning and evaluation efforts at more local levels. The more powerful and specialized medical groups will be free to continue consuming more and more resources for highly specialized equipment and beds, undermining the possible benefits of integrated primary care. Until the specialized medical interests lose their "sacred cow" status, spending for the planning, delivery, and evaluation of coordinated primary care will depend on the leadership of the categorical federal programs who have a vision of larger benefits.

If money, control, and leadership for human services are shifted to the states, the direction in which President Reagan's policy seems to be headed, the federal role in evaluation may become more clearly focused on specialized research and routine monitoring. If funds for the Mental Health Systems Act are appropriated by Congress and block grants to states are not implemented, then federal categorical agencies such as NIMH will be monitoring "performance contracts" written, with each state receiving funds through the new law. In addition, to answer congressional inquiries with respect to national resources and needs, such agencies will continue to require reporting of minimal statistical data, following a path from the local to the state and national levels. The degree to which such routine monitoring will focus on coordinated care will depend on cooperation at the federal level in the design of reporting systems that monitor cross-categorical movement of patients, staff, or other resources. For example, NIMH has plans to implement a Mental Health Statistical Improvement Program (MHSIP), relying on state- and local-level cooperation to use minimal data sets and standardized definition of data elements. Although this will be a great stride toward unified and simplified data reporting by mental health service providers, the minimum data sets do not directly address the issue of coordinated health and mental health care. The data reporting system currently used by BCHS does little to monitor the primary care center patients' uses of mental health services. The design and implementation of the next generation of monitoring systems will have to address the flow of patients, services, and resources across categorical service settings. Furthermore, at this time there are few indications that "performance standards" and state contracts will demand the delivery of coordinated health and mental health services. Since the interest and ability to set performance standards and collect information are highly correlated with the ability to control the allocation of money, future efforts may shift to the state level.

The Proper Order of Things

The task of evaluating coordinated health and mental health care will not be easy. The potential benefits, however, should stimulate increasing efforts to do so. The old order of things will not change easily. An entrenched categorical system must be confronted with good evidence that integrative approaches have cost-effective outcomes.

The unprecedented reduction in the growth rate of government spending will force a major reexamination of the HHS system. Part of that debate may include a closer look at the costs and inefficiencies of our specialized but fragmented nonsystem. Health promotion will be contrasted with chronic disease treatment. Holistic primary care will be contrasted with specialty care. Patient involvement and education will be contrasted to the unilateral authority of the specialist physician.

The potential for evaluation activities to examine the inefficiencies and ineffectiveness of a categorical, specialty nonsystem are reduced to the extent that the sponsors of evaluation are a part of the categorical framework. Will health service funding agencies sponsor evaluations of specialty care? Will categorical mental health funding agencies dare to shift the focus from a narrow examination of mental health services to a study of mental health services' impact on general health? There is some indication that such questions are intriguing to the categorical agencies. However, the risks and uncertainty of asking such questions make it unlikely that there will soon be any major shifts in how evaluation and research dollars are spent. Government agency administrators find it difficult to implement evaluations that touch on the turf of other government bureaucracies. Cooperative inter-agency planning must precede the implementation of evaluation studies. Such cooperation requires trust and a higher-level authority that sanctions such studies. Currently, both are in short supply.

We began this chapter by raising significant questions. Certainly we have not succeeded in answering most of them. The framework we have presented serves only to raise a whole new set of questions. In some ways, we feel we are as confused as ever; but we feel we are confused on a higher level and about more important issues.

References

Broskowski, A., & Attkisson, C. C. *Information systems for health and human services.* New York: Academic Press, in press.

John, D. *Managing the human service system: What have we learned from services integration?* Human Services Monograph Series, No. 4, Project SHARE. Rockville, MD: National Institute of Mental Health, 1977.

Rabkin, E. S., & Silverman, E. M. Passing gas. *Human Nature,* 2, 51-55.

Siegel, L. M., Attkisson, C. C., & Carson, L. Need identification and program planning in the community context. In C. C. Attkisson et al. (Eds.), *Evaluation of human service programs.* New York: Academic Press, 1978.

14

Reducing Medical Costs Through Mental Health Treatment

Research Problems and Recommendations

Emily Mumford
Herbert J. Schlesinger
University of Colorado School of Medicine
Gene V Glass
University of Colorado, School of Education

An enormous literature suggests that emotional factors may play a role in disease processes and in treatment. Disease may be caused or aggravated by emotional distress; emotions can influence the body's ability to recover from illness and surgery; a patient's emotional responses to illness may influence both the doctor's decisions about medical treatment and the way the patient cares for himself—all these have consequences for the course of disease, recovery, the maintenance of health and the use of medical services (Schlesinger, Mumford, & Glass, 1980). A high proportion of those who seek attention in medical practices of general practitioners and medical specialists seem to have "nothing organic wrong with them." To the extent that such complaining is not recognized and treated appropriately, it may lead to misutilization and result in repeated visits, unneeded surgical procedures, excessive medication, delay of effective treatment, and the social costs that accompany them. Several authors have reviewed the literature on the effects of mental health treatment or alcohol, drug abuse, and mental health treat-

AUTHORS' NOTE: The work reported here was supported in part by NIMH under Contract No. 278-78-0037(MH) and by a grant from the John D. and Catherine T. MacArthur Foundation.

ment on the utilization of medical care service (Mumford, Schlesinger, & Glass, 1978; Jones & Vischi, 1979).

In this chapter we will summarize these reviews to prepare for a discussion of the range of problems that interfere with determining whether there is a "cost-offset" effect; that is, a lowering of medical care utilization as a consequence of mental health treatment.

While psychotherapy has been widely practiced under various names for millenia, it has the reputation in some quarters of being a vague treatment for vague complaints with no way of determining the necessity of treatment or assessing results. In fact, psychotherapy has been subjected to more controlled experiment and study than have most medical therapies, aside from drugs. One of us with other colleagues (Smith, Glass, & Miller, 1980) reviewed 475 controlled outcome studies of psychotherapy. Controlling for quality of study and other parameters, Smith et al. found that, on the whole, psychotherapy is beneficial. Across all studies, the average person receiving psychotherapy is better off than 80 percent of those in the untreated control groups.

Review of Studies of the Effects of Psychotherapy on Medical Utilization

We will discuss two types of research evidence on the effects of psychotherapy on medical utilization: (1) archival, time-series studies, and (2) controlled clinical experiments. For all of the shortcomings of the archival approach, it has the advantage of "naturalness" and some major sources of bias from intrusive research interventions are avoided. Although controlled clinical experiments may suffer in varying degrees from "reactive" (Campbell & Stanley, 1966) influences resulting from patient and doctor awareness of the research, they may compensate with superior experimental controls.

Archival, Time-Series Studies of the Impact of Psychotherapy on Medical Utilization

Fifteen studies that examined patients' medical records for a period before and after entry into psychotherapy were located in the published and unpublished literature through April 1979. They differ in whether they use control groups, in duration of observation, and in frequency of pre- and posttherapy observation points. In general, the use of well-matched control groups, longer duration of observations, and higher frequency of observation imply higher quality of experimental design.

One important feature of design, however, critically affects interpretation of findings. The distinction between a relative and an absolute time base is crucial in assessing the validity of the evidence. Observations on a "relative" time base are accumulated at points before or after the date when each patient entered therapy. Thus, "one-month pretherapy" might be June 1975 for one person but August 1976 for another. "Absolute time," in contrast, is the same for all persons in the group under observation; for example, in absolute time, one-month pretherapy is April 1977 for each person in the group.

The importance of this distinction derives from the susceptibility of relative time-series to invalidation from the effect of regression to the mean. This "regression effect" causes mischief in time-series quasi-experiments in the following manner: In reaction to the extreme deviation of the curve, the experimenter is prompted to take some action to bring the curve back to a more typical value. In these circumstances, the experimenter is likely to mistake the expected regression effect—that is, the tendency in a series for extreme values to be followed by values closer to the mean—for the effect of his or her own actions. Hence, the fallacy of "reactive intervention" (Glass, Willson, & Gottman, 1975). In regard to the present analysis, suppose an individual monitors his or her states across time. When discomfort reaches an extremely high level, the person might be prompted to seek psychotherapy. The start of therapy might coincide with the expected decline of the discomfort curve and would likely be interpreted by patient and therapist alike as an ameliorative effect of treatment. An alternative explanation of this quick "improvement" is statistical regression; a movement toward the typical level of the series will reliably follow the high or low points in a time-series. If a control group is not matched for the "discomfort" variable with observations accumulated on a relative time base, there would be no comparable expectation for its values to regress toward the mean. The methodological issues of relative versus absolute time loom especially large in view of possible spurts of high utilization around personal crises, such as a death in the family (Parkes, 1970).

"Statistical regression" is, of course, not in itself an explanation. It is an all-purpose, mathematical name for the movement of data values. There is nothing logically inconsistent with the claim that a person's scores regressed statistically and the claim that all the reasons for the change in those scores are known. Typically, however, the many and varied causes of the probabilistic fluctuations of a time-series are unknown and can be regarded as "error."

Table 14.1 summarizes the finding of all 15 studies in comparable terms: Three studies (Goldberg, Krantz, & Locke, 1970; McHugh, Kahn, &

TABLE 14.1 Summary of Findings from Archival Time-Series Analyses of the Effect of Psychotherapy on Medical Utilization

Study:	Measure of Medical Utilization (corrected to annual rate)	Psychotherapy Group						Control Group						Diff. in % change, +favors control group
		N	Time: Relative or Absolute	Pre and Post	Pre Average	Post Average	% Change	N	Time: Relative or Absolute	Pre and Post	Pre Average	Post Average	% Change	
Duehrssen & Jorswiek (1965)	Days hospitalized	125	Relative	5 yr. pre 5 yr. post	5.4	1.0	−81.5	100	Absolute	5 yr. pre 5 yr. post	5.0	4.6	−8.0	−73.5
Cummings & Follette Follette & Cummings (1966, 1967, 1968)	Medical visits	152	Relative	1 yr. pre 5 yr. post	13.5	10.6	−21.5	152	Absolute	1 yr. pre 5 yr. post	11.0	12.3	+11.8	−33.2
Fink & Goldensohn (1969)	Medical visits	112	Relative	1 yr. pre 2 yr. post	10.53	9.52	−10.0	319	Absolute	1 yr. pre 2 yr. post	8.45	8.46	+0.0	−10.0
Kennecott (1975)	Medical costs	150	Relative	6 mo. pre 6 mo. post	$1118.64	$499.44	−55.4	150	Absolute	6 mo. pre 6 mo. post	$435.00	$441.48	+1.5	−56.9
Goldberg et al. (1970)	Medical visits	256	Relative	1 yr. pre 1 yr. post	4.9	3.4	−30.6	---------- NONE ----------						−30.6
Uris (1974)	Medical visits	45	Absolute	1 yr. pre ('69) 1 yr. post ('71) (1970 excluded)	4.2	3.7	−11.9	90	Absolute	1 yr. pre ('69) 1 yr. post ('71) ('70 excluded)	4.1	3.2	−22.0	+10.1
Kogan et al. (1975)	Medical visits	148	Relative	5 yr. pre 2 yr. post	8.5	7.1	−16.5	148	Absolute	5 yr. pre 2 yr. post	4.3	4.1	−4.7	−11.8
Jameson et al. (1976)	Medical costs	120	Relative	2 yr. pre 2 yr. post	$244.80	$110.64	−54.8		Absolute	2 yr. pre 2 yr. post	$616.20	$237.84	−61.4	+6.6
McHugh et al. (1977)	Medical visits	120	Relative	1 yr. pre 1 yr. post	6.7	11.6	+73.1	---------- NONE ----------						+73.1

Study	N						N						
Goldensohn & Fink (1978)	169	Relative	1 yr. pre 1 yr. post	3.8	3.4	−10.5	141	Absolute	1 yr. pre 1 yr. post	4.6	4.8	+4.3	−14.8
Graves & Hastrup (1978)	21	Relative	1 yr. pre 1 yr. post	5.8	3.7	−36.2	42	Absolute	1 yr. pre 1 yr. post	3.5	4.1	−17.1	−19.1
Kessler (1978)	1,155	Relative	2 yr. pre 2 yr. post	6.3	5.8	−7.9	------NONE------						−7.9
Olbrisch (1978)	55	Absolute	3 mo. pre 1 yr. post	21.6*	6.0*	−72.0	55	Absolute	3 mo. pre 1 yr. post	22.8*	6.4*	−72.0	0
Patterson & Bise (1978)	1,000	Relative	6 mo. pre 6 mo. post	7.6	6.2	−18.4	3,000	Absolute	6 mo. pre 6 mo. post	3.6	3.1	−13.9	−4.5
Rosen & Wiens (1980)	308	Relative	1 yr. pre 1 yr. post	5.0	2.9	−42.0	160	Absolute	1 yr. pre 1 yr. post	2.9	2.7	−6.9	−35.1

Medical visits — Goldensohn & Fink (1978)
Medical visits — Graves & Hastrup (1978)
Medical visits — Kessler (1978)
Medical contacts (visits) all types incl. dental, university health ctr. — Olbrisch (1978)
Medical visits — Patterson & Bise (1978)
Outpatient medical visits — Rosen & Wiens (1980)

Heiman, 1977; and Kessler, 1978) did not employ control groups. Their entries in the final column are the difference between pretest and posttest observations, the best estimate of effect in the absence of a control group. Since the most of the pre/post differences for the psychotherapy groups are confounded by the regression (or "reactive intervention") problem, it might be wise to forebear drawing conclusions. However, the hope of salvaging even a tentative finding from all this effort is strong and justifies risks when methodological scruples would permit no conclusions at all.

In most studies inadequacies in design probably favor the psychotherapy group over the control group. Perhaps the only exception is in the McHugh et al. study (1977), with its apparent long-term, upward trends in utilization. *Recognizing, then, that the figures are probably biased in favor of psychotherapy, the average benefit of therapy is about a 13 percent decrease in medical utilization.* The upward trend among the Mexican-Americans studied by McHugh et al. may represent increased attention to health as well as the expectable and even hoped-for rise in utilization when new services are provided to a previously underserved population. If the McHugh study, which was based on new services in a previously underserved area, is eliminated, then the average benefit calculated from the remaining differences in the last column becomes a 19 percent decrease in medical utilization as a result of psychotherapy.

Because of the problems in design of most of these studies, the hypothesis is quite plausible that they reflect no beneficial effect of psychotherapy on medical utilization. It seems highly unlikely that the true benefits exceed the 19 percent estimated decrease in medical utilization obtained by eliminating the McHugh study from Table 14.1. The conclusion can be drawn with confidence that psychotherapy reduces medical utilization by between zero to 19 percent. More careful research is needed to narrow this band of uncertainty.

Jones and Vischi (1979) summarized their review of the literature on the cost-offset effect of mental health treatment as showing a median effect of 20 percent reduction in medical care utilization. The cost-offsets in those studies reporting reductions of medical care costs ranged from 5 to 85 percent.

Controlled, Experimental Studies of
the Effects of Psychotherapy on Medical Utilization

Controlled experiments entail the assignment of patients to two or more different conditions (e.g., psychotherapy versus a wait-list control) and the

subsequent measurement of outcomes from the different conditions. Sufficient controlled, clinical experimental studies suitable for meta-analysis
(Glass, 1977) on the effects of psychotherapy on medical utilization were
found in three areas: alcoholism, asthma, and recovery from surgery. The
details of quantitative reviews of these experiments are presented elsewhere
(Mumford, et al., 1978, Schlesinger et al., 1980).

Effects of Psychotherapy on Asthma

In brief, psychotherapy (primarily behavioral therapies and hypnother-
apy) shows impressively great effect on ameliorating the effects of asthma.
The effects are substantial on the reduction of utilization of direct medical
services; only 23 percent of the therapy subjects used as many medical
services as half the control subjects.

Effects of Psychotherapy on Alcoholism and Drug Abuse

Averaging results across studies of psychological treatment of alcoholism
yields success rates of 51 percent and 33 percent for psychotherapy and
control conditions, respectively. To put these findings into cost-offset terms,
we could conclude that, on the average, 20 hours of psychotherapy produce
18 "successes" (sobriety six months after therapy) out of every 100 persons
treated. The relapse rates suggest that if the benefits of the therapy are to be
sustained, it must be readministered at periodic intervals. Also, the correlation across the 15 studies between the number of hours of therapy and the
differential "success" rate was positive and reasonably large: +.49.

Jones and Vischi (1979) summarized their review of the impact of alcoholism treatment interventions on medical care utilization, or surrogate
measures (e.g., reduction in paid sick days), as "very substantial in all
twelve of the studies." Sick days were reduced between 38 and 47 percent.
Sickness and accident benefits paid reduced from 33 to 48 percent. They also
found 69 percent fewer hospital days, 40 percent fewer outpatient visits, and
reductions of 27 to 48 percent in outpatient and inpatient cost expenditures.

Jones and Vischi (1979) found that the few studies of the impact of drug
abuse rehabilitation treatment pointed to the same type of results that were
found in the review of alcoholism intervention studies.

Effects of Psychologically Informed Intervention
on Patients Recovering from Surgery

We have been able to locate 30 experimental studies that test the effect of
providing emotional support and/or understanding as an adjunct to medi-

cally required care for patients undergoing surgery. The course of recovery was compared with that of a control group of patients not provided the special attention. The circumstances and findings of each study and the problems in analyzing them as a group have been summarized elsewhere (Schlesinger et al., 1980).

A subset of the outcome indicators is particularly important for its cost-offset implications. Fifteen studies reported the amount of time spent in the hospital by the treatment and the control groups. The average difference in days hospitalized for these 15 studies weighted equally or weighted according to the number of patients studied is slightly more than two days in favor of the intervention group. The difference is statistically reliable.

This effect occurs even though the interventions are mostly modest, either educational, emotionally supportive or both, but not tailored to the needs of the individual patient; that is, all patients in the experimental groups received the intervention under study. Two studies that attempted to match the intervention to the patient show that when the coping style of the patient is compatible with the type of support provided, the intervention appeared to be more effective (DeLong, 1971; Kennedy & Bakst, 1966).

Problems Associated with
Estimating the Cost-Offset Effect

Assessing whether there is cost-offset attributable to including a mental health component in primary health care would seem to be a straightforward research problem. Instead, it is encumbered with difficulties from several sources, some conceptual and methodological, others practical and statistical.

First, the very assumption that mental health services should reduce the utilization of other medical services needs to be examined closely. Certainly mental health care should be required to demonstrate that it is effective and even that it is cost-effective, which is to say efficient. But should it have to justify itself by displacing other medical services? There are certain circumstances when such an offset might be expected, chiefly when physical health services are misutilized and overutilized—that is, substituted for unavailable, inaccessible, or inconceivable mental health care.

The reasoning underlying this expectation is that people will seek help for emotional problems whether or not a proper channel is provided. Emotional problems frequently have somatic components, and it is easier for many people to ask for medical attention for sleeplessness, "tension," low back pain, or G.I. disturbance rather than for "depression."

The Appropriateness of Utilization

Reducing misutilization must be part of any attempt to improve health service systems. But misutilization may coincide with either *under*utilization or *over*utilization. Self-neglect or abuse is common among the emotionally ill, a factor which may contribute to the excess morbidity and mortality from physical disease noted among psychiatric patients (Mumford et al., 1978; Hankin & Oktay, 1979; Goldberg, Comstock, & Hornstra, 1979). One effect of successful mental health intervention for such persons should be to *increase* medical utilization (Borus, Burns, Jacobson, Macht, Morrill, & Wilson, 1979). For example, services are misutilized and underutilized by parents who fail to bring a child to medical care even though a reversible disease process has been identified through an expensive screening program. Services are misutilized and eventually overutilized when preventive services are not used and avoidable illness results in hospitalization. Misutilization also occurs when neglect of prenatal care contributes to unnecessary complications at delivery or to the birth of a defective child. Recognizing the paradox that failure to use medical services can result in overuse and misuse of health services is central to many preventive efforts and health education campaigns. The time, money, and health potential wasted when medical advice is sought but ignored is the subject of a burgeoning literature on "compliance" with medical advice (Barofsky, 1977; Sackett & Haynes, 1976).

Excessive utilization directly raises costs of medical service. But it is also of great concern to physicians because it may reflect inappropriate utilization and hence lower quality of medical care—ironically, at higher expense. Physicians, patients, and third-party payers share an interest in realizing an optimal level of medical utilization that results in improved functioning with a minimum of unnecessary procedures, visits, and hospitalizations.

Health Versus Mental Health

A second conceptual problem is the supposed distinction between *mental* health care and *physical* health care. While conceptually distinguishable, emotional and physical distress are so inextricably intertwined that it can be counterproductive to encourage treatment of physical malfunction while discouraging treatment of emotional malfunction. Furthermore, the strategies that would be required to assign patients to services treating *only* psychological disorders or *only* physical disorders boggle the mind in light of the many studies that demonstrate the coexistence of both kinds of problems (Mumford et al., 1978; Hankin & Oktay, 1979).

Definitional Difficulties

A third conceptual problem has to do with the very nature of the major variables of interest. Health itself, which is the prime outcome variable, is largely represented in research by medical utilization, a presumed negative indicator. Often the definition of health and whether an emotional problem is "a problem in living," a religious problem, an ethical problem, a social problem, or a medical problem seems to depend on whose purse is being gored. Medical utilization is often chosen as the indicator of convenience. It is not a simple variable, but rather a congeries of hospital days, doctor visits, procedures done, and medicine prescribed. Since it is expressible in dollars spent, it is a convenient way to refer to the output of a health services system.

But there are other "hard," or easy to measure, indicators, and any number of "soft" ones that could be considered. "Soft" indicators generally refer to subjective issues, feeling well or ill, satisfied with medical services or not. While more difficult to measure, they may be equally or even more important as are the "hard" ones to the persons who are the patients of these studies, as well as to society.

Notwithstanding all these caveats, it is important for planning health care systems to know if providing mental health services has any effect on the utilization of other medical services. While we focus here on the influence of psychotherapeutic intervention, medical utilization is also influenced by a wide range of psychosocial, economic, geographic, and financial factors (Engel, 1977a, 1977b; Lipowski, 1975, 1977; Glass, 1977; Fabrega, 1975; Kaplan, 1975; Mechanic, 1976). We list some of these in order to warn the reader about the complexity of the field. Among the factors to which medical utilization is sensitive are the following:

(1) The tendency in our society to "medicalize" life problems; the "selling of medicine" as holding the key to health, happiness, sexual success, and social popularity (Aday & Andersen, 1978; Eisenberg, 1977).

(2) Perceptions of health—emotional and physical—and the place of health in hierarchies of values (Kaminsky & Slavney, 1976; Lesse, 1974).

(3) Perceptions of "rights"—to care, concern, treatment equality, attention—all expressible as "the right to treatment" (Mumford, 1977).

(4) Secondary gain—the use of the experience of complaint of illness and medical attention to legitimatize a wish to be cared for, to be excused from fulfilling obligations and responsibilities, to fulfill a desire for "compensation" either for actual disability or for a sense of being treated unfairly by life (Mechanic, 1976; Dohrenwend & Dohrenwend, 1969).

(5) Economic conditions. It has been observed that visits to physicians and rates of hospitalization increase in times of economic decline (Brenner, 1973).

(6) Availability of health services—including geographic factors, clinic and office hours, presence of emergency services or walk-in services, financial conditions, and social and cultural expectations and patterns of help-seeking of the "patient" population (Mechanic, 1976; Clancy & Gove, 1974; Webb, Thompson, & Whitt, 1977).

(7) Stress and "life events" may lead to emotional distress presenting as physical disease. Emotional distress, etc. may also affect existing disease, exacerbating symptoms or affecting the body directly or indirectly. Emotional factors, etc. may also trigger visits to physicians for a previously ignored physical illness (Mechanic, 1972; Fontana, Dowds, Marcus, & Rakusin, 1976; Roghmann & Haggerty, 1972).

(8) Physical illness may itself lead to social and/or psychological problems, including family disruption, which in turn may lead to emotional distress further aggravating the physical illness and leaving the patient dependent on medical facilities (Rappaport, 1975; Engel, 1977b; Gersten, Langer, Eisenberg, & Simcha-Fagan, 1977).

(9) Patterns of response to medical advice resulting from the nature of care given and the setting in which it is given, as well as cultural factors and personal idiosyncracies (Barofsky, 1977; Becker & Maiman, 1975; Sackett & Haynes, 1976; Rosenberg & Raynes, 1976; Stimson & Webb, 1975).

(10) Professional convictions of health care providers about the appropriate "treatment" of complaints presented to them (e.g., surgeons tend to recommend surgery; see Lawson & Jick, 1976; Sedgewick, 1974; Vayda, 1973; Bunker, 1970).

(11) Economic motives of health care providers (Fuchs, 1974).

(12) Iatrogenic illness (Bercel, 1968; Fuchs, 1974; Reidenberg, 1968; Ogilvie and Ruedy, 1967).

(13) Risk-taking behavior—smoking, overeating, lack of exercise, careless driving, etc. (Pomerleau, Bass, & Crown, 1975; Singer, Garfinkel, Cohen, & Srole, 1976).

(14) Environmental conditions—pollution, unsafe industrial conditions, traffic hazards, etc. (Fuchs, 1974).

(15) The nature and effectiveness of social controls over availability of health care and its utilization (Goshen, 1963; McCarthy & Widmer, 1974).

This list is not exhaustive, and many of the factors can be further subdivided. Since medical utilization is sensitive to so many factors, it would be all the more noteworthy if the availability and use of psychotherapy or other forms of "mental health," or psychologically-informed, intervention can be shown to influence it.

Psychotherapy is also a complex variable subject to multiple influences. To summarize, one must consider:

(1) the kind of psychotherapy offered. Psychotherapies are classifiable in terms of the unit treated (e.g., individual or group, couples or family), in terms of the theory that inspires the effort, defines the presumed mechanisms or processes, and explains the results.

(2) the time dimension of psychotherapy. How frequently is the patient seen for sessions of what length and over what period, intermittently or continuously? Long duration of treatment and high frequency of sessions are sometimes considered to guarantee "intensivity," while a brief episode or infrequent visits of psychotherapy may be dismissed as "superficial." These appellations may not be justified.

(3) Therapies are not always conducted in a "pure" form but may be combined with each other as well as with other means of providing social support, and with medication.

(4) The quality of the psychotherapy given. Even more difficult than knowing precisely what occurs between therapist and patient is knowing how representative the therapy is of what it was supposed to be, and how well it was done. In addition to the barrier of patient privacy, the conceptual tools for evaluating diverse therapies directly are rudimentary.

Again, since psychotherapy and medical utilization are each complex and messy variables, these complexities, if they could be assumed to vary randomly, might be expected to wash out any true relationships that more refined studies might reveal. Thus, if studies conducted at the present state of the art reliably show a relationship, they would argue for remarkably robust effects.

Methodological Problems

In addition to conceptual and philosophical issues there are methodological problems besetting utilization research that make it difficult to estimate cost-offsets precisely. First, most of the research is clinical. Patients are seen in naturalistic settings where treatment conditions cannot generally be manipulated to achieve experimental cleanliness. In clinical research we know that "the intervention" is not the only variable at work. A multifactorial approach is needed, but rarely are there sufficient patients and sufficiently controlled conditions. More important, all the factors that operate in the field have not yet been identified clearly. Second, much of the research in the field has been archival, or retrospective, making use of existing data gathered for purposes other than research.

A third issue, the problem of selecting appropriate control groups, has flawed many studies in the field, in ways we indicated earlier. A fourth issue is the time when one should assess the outcome of psychological intervention. Should it be directly at the end of treatment or a month, a year, or a decade later?

While these multiple difficulties could lead one to conclude that research in this field is all but impossible, much work has actually been done, as we reviewed in the earlier section of this chapter. Through continued research efforts these problems can be addressed and solved.

Summary

A review of the problems in determining whether a cost-offset by reducing medical care utilization can be expected from mental health treatment shows that the difficulties are conceptual and methodological as well as practical and statistical. The problems are difficult to solve but not insurmountable.

Most of the archival studies of the effects of psychotherapy on medical utilization are flawed by problems of experimental design. A critical, quantitative review of these studies indicates a likely reduction of between zero and 19 percent in medical utilization and costs.

A quantitative review of controlled, experimental studies assessing the effects of various kinds of psychotherapy on alcoholism and asthma show positive effects on outcome indicators with clear implications for a significant and sizable cost-offset. A similar review of studies of the effects of "psychologically informed" intervention on patients recovering from surgery shows a clear cost-offset resulting from a more than two-day-shorter hospital stay for the intervention group.

Quite aside from the intrinsic value of offering specific care for patient's emotional problems and humane and considerate care for their medical and surgical problems, the evidence is that providing psychotherapy and psychologically informed care can be cost-effective and that a cost-offset may result from the inclusion of a mental health component in primary care systems.

References

Aday, L., & Andersen, R. America's health care system: A comprehensive portrait. *Robert Wood Johnson Foundation Special Report,* No. 1, pp. 4-15. City: Publisher, 1978.

Barofsky, I. (Ed.). *Medication compliance.* Thorofare, NJ: Charles B. Slack, 1977.

Becker, M. N., & Maiman, L. A. Sociobehavioral determinants of compliance with health and medical care recommendations. *Medical Care,* 1975, 13, 109-124.

Bercel, N. A. Concluding remarks. *Diseases of the Nervous System,* 1968, 29 (Supplement), 77-78.

Borus, J. F., Burns, B. J., Jacobson, A. M., Macht, L. B., Morrill, R. G., & Wilson, E. M. Neighborhood health centers as providers of coordinated mental health care. Background paper for Invitational Conference on the Provision of Mental Health Services in Primary Care Settings, April 2-3, 1979.

Brenner, H. *Mental illness and the economy.* Cambridge, MA: Harvard University Press, 1973.

Budman, S. H., Wertlieb, D., Budman, S., & Demby, A. Maximizing the offset of medical utilization via psychological services: A strategy for intervention. Paper presented at the National Institute of Mental Health, April 5, 1979.

Bunker, J. P. Surgical manpower, a comparison of operations and surgeons in the United States and in England and Wales. *New England Journal of Medicine,* 1970, 282, 135-144.

Campbell, D. T., & Stanley, J. C. *Experimental and quasi-experimental designs for research.* Chicago: Rand McNally, 1966.

Clancy, K., & Gove, W. Sex differences in mental illness: An analysis of response bias in self reports. *American Journal of Sociology,* 1974, 80, 205-216.

Cummings, N. A., & Follette, W. T. Psychiatric services and medical utilization in a prepaid health plan setting. Part II. *Medical Care,* 1968, 6, 31-41.

DeLong, R. D. Individual differences in patterns of anxiety arousal, stress-relevant information and recovery from surgery. *Dissertation Abstracts International,* 1971, 32, 554B-555B.

Dohrenwend, B. P., & Dohrenwend, B. S. *Social status and psychological disorder.* New York: John Wiley, 1969.

Duehrssen, A., & Jorswiek, E. An empirical and statistical inquiry into the therapeutic potential of psychoanalytic treatment. *Der Nervenarzt,* 1965, 36, 166-169.

Eisenberg, L. Disease and illness. *Culture Medicine and Psychiatry,* 1977, 1, 9-23.

Engel, G. The need for a new medical model: A challenge for biomedicine. *Science,* 1977, 196, 129-136. (a)

Engel, G. Emotional stress and sudden death. *Psychology Today,* 1977, 11, 114-118; 153-154. (b)

Fabrega, H. The position of psychiatry in the understanding of human disease. *Archives of General Psychiatry,* 1975, 32, 1500-1512.

Fink, R., & Goldensohn, S. S. Psychiatric treatment and patterns of medical care. Unpublished report to NIMH, 1969, No. 7169, pp. 33-51.

Follette, W., & Cummings, N. Psychiatric services and medical utilization in a prepaid health plan setting. *Medical Care,* 1967, 5, 25-35.

Fontana, A. F., Dowds, B. N., Marcus, J. D., & Rakusin, J. M. Coping with interpersonal conflicts through life events and hospitalization. *Journal of Nervous and Mental Disease,* 1976, 162, 88-98.

Fuchs, V. R. *Who shall live?* New York: Basic Books, 1974.

Gersten, J. C., Langer, T. S., Eisenberg, J. G., & Simcha-Fagan, O. An evaluation of the etiologic role of stressful life-change events in psychological disorder. *Journal of Health and Social Behavior,* 1977, 18, 228-244.

Glass, D. C. *Behavior patterns, stress and coronary disease.* Hillsdale, NJ: Lawrence Erlbaum, 1977.

Glass, G. V Summarizing effect sizes. *New Directions for Methodology of Social and Behavioral Science,* 1980, 5, 13-31.

Glass, G. V, Willson, V. L., & Gottman, J. M. *Design and analysis of time-series experiments.* Boulder: Colorado Associated University Press, 1975.

Goldberg, E. L., Comstock, G. W., & Hornstra, R. K. Depressed mood and subsequent physical illness. *American Journal of Psychiatry,* 1979, 136, 530-534.

Goldberg, I. D., Krantz, G., & Locke, B. Z. Effects of a short-term outpatient psychiatric therapy benefit on the utilization of medical services in a prepaid group practice medical program. *Medical Care,* 1970, 8, 419-428.

Goldensohn, S. S., & Fink, R. Mental health services for Medicaid enrollees in a prepaid group practice (HMO). Paper presented at the 131st Annual Meeting of the American Psychiatric Association, Atlanta, Georgia, May 11, 1978.

Goshen, C. E. The high cost of nonpsychiatric care. *General Practitioner,* 1963, 27, 227-235.

Graves, R., & Hastrup, J. Effects of psychological treatment on medical utilization in a multidisciplinary health clinic for low income minority children. Paper presented at the annual Southwestern Psychological Association meeting, New Orleans, Louisiana, April 1978.

Hankin, J., & Oktay, J. S. *Mental disorder and primary medical care: An analytic review of the literature.* NIMH Monograph Series D, No. 5. DHEW Publication No. (ADM) 78-661. Washington, DC: Government Printing Office, 1979.

Jameson, J., Shuman, L. J., & Young, W. W. The effects of outpatient psychiatric utilization on the costs of providing third-party coverage. Research Series 18, Blue Cross of Western Pennsylvania, December 1976, pp. 1-38.

Jones, K., & Vischi, T. Impact of alcohol, drug abuse and mental health treatment on medical care utilization. A review of the literature. *Medical Care,* 1980, 17 (Supplement).

Kaminsky, M. J., & Slavney, P. R. Methodology and personality in Briquet's Syndrome: A reappraisal. *American Journal of Psychiatry,* 1976, 133, 85-88.

Kaplan, H. B. Understanding the social and social-psychological antecedents and consequences of psychopathology: A review of reports of invitational conferences. *Journal of Health and Social Behavior,* 1975, 16, 135-151.

Kennecott Copper Corporation. *Insight. A program for troubled people.* Salt Lake City: Utah Copper Division, 1975.

Kennedy, J. A., & Bakst, H. The influence of emotions on the outcome of cardiac surgery: A predictive study. *Bulletin of the New York Academy of Medicine,* 1966, 42, 811-849.

Kessler, L. Episodes of psychiatric care and medical utilization in a prepaid group practice. Doctor of science dissertation, Johns Hopkins University School of Hygiene and Public Health, Baltimore, Maryland, May 1978.

Kogan, W. S., Thompson, D. J., Brown, J. R., & Newman, H. F. Impact of integration of mental health service and comprehensive medical care. *Medical Care,* 1975, 13, 934-943.

Lawson, D. H., & Jick, H. Drug prescribing in hospitals: An international comparison. *American Journal of Public Health,* 1976, 66, 644-648.

Lesse, S. *Masked depression.* New York: Jason Aronson, 1974.

Lipowski, Z. J. Psychiatry of somatic diseases: Epidemiology, pathogenesis, classification. *Comprehensive Psychiatry,* 1975, 16, 105-124.

Lipowski, Z. J. Psychosomatic medicine in the seventies: An overview. *American Journal of Psychiatry,* 1977, 134, 233-244.

McCarthy, E. G., & Widmer, G. W. Effects of screening by consultants on recommended elective surgical procedures. *New England Journal of Medicine,* 1974, 291, 1331-1335.

McHugh, J. P., Kahn, M. W., & Heiman, E. Relationships between mental health treatment and medical utilization among low-income Mexican-American patients: Some preliminary findings. *Medical Care,* 1977, 15, 439-444.

Mechanic, D. Social-psychologic factors affecting the presentation of bodily complaints. *New England Journal of Medicine,* 1972, 286, 1132-1139.

Mechanic, D. Sociocultural and socio-psychological factors affecting personal responses to psychological disorder. *Journal of Health and Social Behavior,* 1975, 16, 393-404.

Mechanic, D. *The growth of bureaucratic medicine.* New York: John Wiley, 1976.

Mumford, E. Culture: Life perspectives and the social meanings of illness. In R. Simons & H. Pardes (Eds.), *Understanding human behavior in health and illness.* Baltimore: Williams and Wilkins, 1977.

Mumford, E., Schlesinger, H. J., & Glass, G. V A critical review and indexed bibliography of the literature up to 1978 on the effects of psychotherapy on medical utilization. Report to NIMH, Contract No. 278-78-0049(MH). Rockville, Maryland, 1978.

Mumford, E., Schlesinger, H. J., & Glass, G. V Problems of analyzing the cost offset of including a mental health component in primary care. In *Mental health services in general health care, vol. 1.* Washington, DC: Institute of Medicine, National Academy of Sciences, 1979.

Olbrisch, M. E. Evaluation of a stress management program for high utilizers of a prepaid university health service. Ph.D. dissertation, Department of Psychology, Florida State University, August 1978.

Ogilvie, R. I., & Ruedy, J. Adverse drug reactions during hospitalization. *Canadian Medical Association Journal,* 1967, 97, 1450-1457.

Parkes, C. M. The first year of bereavement: A longitudinal study of the reaction of London widows to the death of their husbands. *Psychiatry,* 1970, 33, 444-467.

Patterson, D., & Bise, B. Report pursuant to NIMH Contract No. 282-77-0219(MS), January 1978.

Pomerleau, O., Bass, F., & Crown, V. Role of behavior modification in preventive medicine. *New England Journal of Medicine,* 1975, 292, 1277-1282.

Rappaport, M. Medically oriented psychiatry: An approach to improving the quality of mental health care. *Hospital and Community Psychiatry,* 1975, 26, 811-815.

Regier, D. A., Goldberg, I. D., Burns, B. J., Hankin, J., Hoeper, E. W., & Nycz, G. R. Epidemiological and health services research findings in four organized health/mental health service settings. Paper presented at the ADAMHA Health Maintenance Organization Conference, November 30, 1977.

Reidenberg, M. M. Registry of adverse drug reactions. *Journal of the American Medical Association,* 1968, 203, 85-88.

Roghmann, K. J., & Haggerty, R. J. Family stress and the use of health services. *International Journal of Epidemiology,* 1972, 1, 279-286.

Rosen, J. C., & Wiens, A. N. On psychological intervention and medical services utilization. *American Psychologist,* 1980, 35, 761-762.

Rosenberg, C. M., & Raynes, A. E. *Keeping patients in psychiatric treatment.* Cambridge, MA: Ballinger, 1976.

Sackett, D. L., & Haynes, R. B. *Compliance with therapeutic regimens.* Baltimore: Johns Hopkins University Press, 1976.

Schlesinger, H. J., Mumford, E., & Glass, G. V The effects of psychological intervention on recovery from surgery. In F. Guerra & J. A. Aldrete (Eds.), *Emotional and psychological responses to anesthesia and surgery.* New York: Grune and Stratton, 1980.

Sedgewick, P. Medical individualism. *Hastings Center Studies,* 1974, 2, 69-80.

Singer, E., Garfinkel, R., Cohen, S. M., & Srole, L. Mortality and mental health: Evidence from the Midtown Manhattan restudy. *Social Science and Medicine,* 1976, 10, 517-525.

Smith, M. L., Glass, G. V, & Miller, T. I. *Benefits of psychotherapy.* Baltimore: Johns Hopkins University Press, 1980.

Stimson, G., & Webb, G. *Going to see the doctor.* London: Routledge & Kegan Paul, 1975.

Uris, J. S. Effects of medical utilization and diagnosis on general medical care utilization in a prepaid clinic setting. Report by Western Interstate Commission on Higher Education (WICHE) Intern, Boulder, Colorado, 1974.

Vayda, E. A comparison of surgical rates in Canada and in England and Wales. *New England Journal of Medicine,* 1973, 289, 1224-1229.

Webb, S. B., Jr., Thompson, J. D., & Whitt, I. B. Statewide trends in emergency department utilization. *Inquiry,* 1977, 14, 402-408.

15

Behavioral Emergencies in Medical Settings

Elinor Walker

U.S. Department of Health and Human Services

What is a Behavioral Emergency?

The emergency physician, that new medical specialist who must also be a generalist, is trained to deal with acute conditions during the period when time is a critical dimension of care. Emergency medical care generally involves stabilization and appropriate referral for definitive care. The term "behavioral emergency" reflects this perspective and is consistent with the growth of emergency medical services (EMS) systems. An organized EMS system tends to sort patients by symptoms and to group the most critically ill or injured patients into broad categories which indicate the specialty care required. These categories are set out in federal law (EMS Systems Act of 1973—PL 93-154) and regulation as "cardiac," "trauma," "burn," "poisoning," "high-risk perinatal," "spinal cord," and "behavioral" emergencies.

The category "behavioral emergency" usually includes psychiatric and substance-abuse events; but the boundaries are murky. For example, an attempted suicide is called a behavioral emergency, but attempted suicide

---

AUTHOR'S NOTE: This chapter has developed from experience in the emergency medical services research program of the National Center for Health Services Research, under the leadership of Lawrence R. Rose, M.D., who stimulated the ideas contained herein. Dr. Rose also reviewed and edited the paper, removing many imprecisions and inelegancies. The views expressed are those of the author, and no official endorsement by the National Center for Health Services Research is intended or should be inferred. The federal government may reproduce and distribute this material royalty-free provided the publisher's copyright is prominently acknowledged.

involving a drug overdose is just as likely to be counted as a poisoning. An abused child is probably recorded as trauma; the person with the behavioral problem, the abuser, may not be encountered by the emergency system at all. A head injury victim may be judged to be a patient with disordered behavior. EMS systems are expected to recognize and provide initial management for these kinds of emergencies and to refer them to an appropriate source of definitive care as necessary.

The Emergency Medical Services Systems Act defined an EMS system as a comprehensive, integrated system comprised of 15 components:

(1) trained personnel;

(2) training programs for personnel;

(3) a central communications system with a single telephone number for access, such as "9-1-1";

(4) transportation facilities;

(5) institutional facilities, classified according to the level of care available;

(6) special care units;

(7) coordinated public safety agencies;

(8) opportunity for participation of residents in policy formation;

(9) provision of emergency care regardless of ability to pay;

(10) provision for referral of patients to follow-up and rehabilitation;

(11) a record system in which a patient's records are linked to permit audit of care throughout the emergency phase;

(12) public education and information on how to use the emergency system;

(13) review and evaluation of the EMS system;

(14) a plan for delivering emergency care in disasters; and

(15) reciprocal aid agreements among neighboring systems.

An important attribute of an EMS system is its *regional* character; the Department of Health and Human Services has divided the country for EMS purposes into 304 regions which can compete for federal funds. The funds are not provided for day-to-day operations, nor, in most cases, to buy equipment. Instead, they provide support to a single organizational entity in each region which proposes to coordinate existing services and providers and thereby to establish or improve a comprehensive, integrated EMS system.

Problems in Care of Behavioral Emergencies

Another facility responsible for providing care to patients with mental health emergencies is the Community Mental Health Center (CMHC). Catchment areas for CMHCs do not necessarily correspond geographically with EMS regions, and in most ways the systems operate with little or no relationship to each other. Even when the CMHC is closely tied to the emergency department, managers and staff do not seem to appreciate their relationships to the EMS system. Under the Community Mental Health Systems Act, which authorizes federal support of CMHCs, 24-hour emergency care is one of the services that must be provided. A few years ago, however, a surveyor attempted to reach the emergency service of each of a sample of CMHCs outside regular working hours. About a third of the time no one answered the telephone, or the answer was a recorded message with no provision for further communication (Jacobs, 1977). Although a later survey (Psychiatric News, 1977) showed improvements, the emergency service often is nothing more than a telephone operator, with rotating staff members "on call." It appears that the mental health system may not be well organized to respond to unscheduled events, especially if they occur at night or on weekends.

The EMS system, on the other hand, is designed to deal with unscheduled events but is not comfortable in managing "behavioral emergencies." People whose behavior is disordered, bizarre, hysterical, or socially undesirable tend to produce feelings of uneasiness, fear, or resentment in emergency department personnel. Patients who are known to present frequently for "drying out" or for minor complaints with no apparent physical basis also create staff hostility. Chronic mental patients, alcoholics, drug addicts, the homeless, and other "down-and-out" populations are often labeled "GO-MERS," short for "Get out of my emergency room."

Most sizable emergency departments have some relationship with a psychiatric service. Frequently a CMHC is located on-site at a hospital, and the two services provide backup to each other. In other settings a particular psychiatric unit with mental health professionals is responsible for supporting the emergency physician or nurse. Often, however, this apparent coordination masks serious deficiencies in care. One psychiatrist told of receiving a call from the emergency department to come and take care of a catatonic patient. When he arrived he found that in fact the patient was dead (Hall, 1980). A patient who arrives at an emergency department without an obvious medical or surgical disease, whose behavior suggests a psychiatric episode, may not receive an adequate medical workup before a psychiatric consultation is requested; this "consult" often amounts to "dumping"—the emergency physician may not participate further in the management of that patient. The consulting psychiatrist, on the other hand, may assume that physical diseases have been ruled out by adequate examination. The potential for missing a serious illness is great, and the problem occurs with some frequency. Development of emergency medicine as a specialty, requiring some training in behavioral problems, and development of the new subspecialty of emergency psychiatry may offer a prospect of better care for such patients (Barry, Kharabi, Nyman, & Schmidt, 1979; Fauman, 1979).

Other problems come about because of community pressures. A troublesome example is the dilemma facing the physician who must care for a patient whose behavioral disorder represents a danger to self or others, such as one who has attempted suicide or threatened violence against another. Almost every state has provisions for confining such a person for some brief period of time for observations and/or treatment. But such confinement, when it is involuntary, conflicts with basic civil liberties, and is the subject of continuing struggle in the courts. In California, the law provides that a 72-hour involuntary commitment is permissible after certification by a psychiatrist; psychiatrists who certify, however, face later hearings and become vulnerable to litigation. On the other hand, the potentially dangerous patient who is released and goes on to fulfill that potential creates enormous resentment against psychiatry and even perhaps the entire medical profession. In any case, EMS personnel are used to dealing with persons who seek help or are in no condition to refuse it; the "involuntary" patient is an exceptionally difficult problem for them, especially in pre-hospital care situations.

Failure to provide adequate emergency medical care to the alcoholic or the drug abuser can result in death; and failure to refer a substance abuser to an adequate source of definitive therapy represents poor medical management, to say the least. Scarcity of resources, lack of awareness of resources that do exist, or hostile attitudes on the part of EMS workers interfere with effective performance in this area.

Deficiencies of these kinds represent real and potential dangers to the health of patients and the well-being of the community. Other problems are less obvious but equally important. For example, it is a matter of medical folklore that many people who repeatedly seek medical care for minor illnesses are probably more in need of mental health care. Other patients who exhibit bizarre or disruptive behavior may be "deinstitutionalized" chronic mental patients in crisis. The management of such patients by emergency departments or pre-hospital care personnel probably tends to be both ineffective and inefficient and represents a heavy burden upon emergency department resources as well as on the health care system generally. Estimates vary, but some 30 percent of emergency department patients may fall into the category "behavioral emergency," and these patients may take up as much as 50 percent of provider time in management (Barton, 1979).

Such problems provide opportunities to use research methods to determine the performance of the system in providing emergency care to the behavioral patient. With adequate methods for measuring system performance, it is then possible to design policies which are likely to improve effectiveness or efficiency, or both. A plausible strategy for such research, based upon experience with research in care of cardiac, trauma, and other emergencies over the past six years, is presented below.

Research in EMS System Effectiveness in Care of Behavioral Emergencies

Despite many years of conceptual and methodologic progress in evaluative research in health and mental health care, most programs are still evaluated only at the level of patients-per-resource-unit, with little or no attention paid to quality issues. Quality-of-care research has improved enormously in recent years; yet most health and mental health quality appraisal consists, at best, of little more than case review against implicit standards. Where attempts are made to compare one program against another in order to develop reimbursement standards or to make other policy decisions, there is little effort to control for case-mix. Virtually nowhere is the care of behavioral emergencies in medical settings subjected to any systematic quality appraisal method.

Considerations or comparisons of the cost-effectiveness of health or mental health programs are obviously impossible in the absence of measures of effectiveness; such discussions are not merely frivolous but even perhaps dangerous. In the absence of quality standards, pressures to increase "productivity" have an all-too-predictable result, but the increasing scarcity of funds is forcing decisions based upon whatever measures are available.

The ultimate effectiveness measure, of course, centers on the outcome of the care to the patient:[1] a change in health (or mental health) status that can be related to the care received. Emergency care of any injury or illness is exceptionally difficult to relate to a change in health status. One reason for this is that much of the care delivered in an emergency medical setting is not for the most serious conditions, but is in fact ambulatory care for relatively minor and nonurgent problems.[2] In many instances, the conditions are self-limiting, and the likelihood of a really bad or really good outcome does not depend on the quality of care. The truly serious conditions, in which outcomes can be measured readily in terms of survival or meaningful reduction of morbidity, are relatively infrequent. This is probably as much the case in mental health as in physical health care. Thus, measuring change in health status is a difficult problem in terms of discriminating often subtle changes in large numbers of patients or achieving sufficient numbers of patients with dramatic changes.

Apart from measurement, there are other difficulties related to inferring that any differences in outcome one can find are attributable to the care received, especially the emergency care received. The cases whose outcomes are most susceptible to measurement often undergo rather long and complex courses of care, of which the emergency portion is only the beginning. It is necessary, then, either to control for the influence of the care received after the patient leaves the emergency department or to estimate "outcome" on the basis of data available at the point when the emergency care ends—a "proximate outcome."

An even more important problem relates to case-mix. Attempts have been made in emergency care research to compare outcomes for one kind of emergency versus another. For example, in Tucson, a study (Buck, Brimmer, & Putzier, 1976) compared outcomes of patients who received prehospital care from "paramedics" with those who arrived at the emergency department some other way. The results showed outcomes to be worse for the group that had been treated and transported by the paramedics. Paramedics are emergency medical technicians (EMTs) who have received up to 2000 hours of training in advanced life support (ALS), which includes such procedures as esophageal intubation, placing intravenous lines, and administering certain drugs. They staff vehicles equipped with expensive communication equipment which permits two-way voice contact with a physician at a base hospital and often includes telemetric transmission of physiologic data, including EKG signals. An ALS system is expensive; and therefore it would be useful to determine whether it makes a difference. If it is unlikely that paramedics are killing people, the most plausible explanation for the Tucson results is that the sicker people are more likely to receive ALS, and are also more likely to have bad outcomes. Case-mix is the problem here, and the customary three-category, ordinal measure of severity (emergent, urgent, nonurgent) is insensitive to the variations that make a difference in emergency care.

At this point, it is perhaps useful to consider the current state of the art in measurement of outcomes of mental health care. A variety of outcome measures is available, many of which were tested in outpatient settings. The Urban Institute (Schainblatt, 1977) has prepared a rather thorough discussion of ways to monitor outcomes of mental health treatment programs. A conceptual framework is available for developing strategies for mental health quality assessment in relationship to "medical" care and what has been done in medical care quality assessment (Brook, Avery, Greenfield, Harris, Lelah, Solomon, & Ware, 1979). Global assessment scaling (Newman, Burwell, & Underhill, 1978), goal-attainment scaling (Kiresuk & Sherman, 1968), the SCL-90 (Derogatis, Rickels, & Rock, 1975), quality-of-life measures (Bigelow, Brodsky, & Hallgren, 1978; Ciarlo & Reihman, 1974), and some others have been found to be reasonably reliable and sensitive to changes over the course of care. None seems to have been tested with emergency patients; nor, so far as this writer is aware, has there been much use of experimental or quasi-experimental design in an attempt to attribute these changes to the care itself. Improvement over time is a characteristic of many self-limiting conditions, and only a careful design can eliminate this and other competing explanations for change in status. A serious source of difficulty is the lack of uniformity in the care received. When you do not know who is doing what to whom, it is unlikely that you will observe interpretable differences in outcome, and certainly you will not be able to produce credible recommendations concerning policies or operating procedures.

What is to be done, then, to provide administrators, clinicians, planners, and other decision makers with information they can use to improve the care of behavioral emergencies? The experience from the program in emergency medical services research, administered since 1974 by the National Center for Health Services Research, appears to offer the basis for a research strategy, though almost none of this work has dealt with behavioral emergencies.

A Framework for Evaluation Research

Classifying the Patient

In the area of emergency care, the measurement of case-mix must be two-dimensional, including both type of condition and immediacy of need for care. (The latter dimension is especially problematic if existing mental-health status measures such as those cited above are applied in an emergency department setting.) Two basic approaches to case-mix measurement have been used (or attempted) in research on cardiac and trauma emergencies: the *severity measure* and the *tracer condition*.

A severity index, or an index of criticality, is a measure of urgency of need for care; it estimates the consequences of failure to meet that need. It can be seen, in effect, as the reciprocal of a health status index. It would be unimportant for evaluating emergency care if enough patients could be randomly assigned to treatment versus control groups, but randomization is seldom possible in situations like this. A good severity index is useful not only for evaluation but also for purposes of triage and for assessing the care given to an individual patient.

Several researchers have undertaken or examined different approaches to developing and testing severity indexes (Champion & Sacco, 1979; Gustafson, 1975; Krischer, 1976). The ideal would be a single index applicable to any emergency condition, including behavioral emergencies, but so far the indexes have had to be condition-specific (i.e., one for burns, one for head injuries, etc.).

If extensive empirical knowledge exists as to the natural history of a disease and the likelihood of a specified outcome, it is fairly easy to translate that information into a severity index. This is seldom the case even for medical conditions, and probably is less so for most behavioral emergencies. There are other ways of approaching the problem, however. Gustafson (1975) tested indices developed from subjective estimates of expert clinicians according to "multi-attribute uility theory." Various techniques exist for achieving consensus estimates of otherwise unknown quantities and have been tested in medical situations (Nutt, 1974; Boone, Young and Associates, 1975).

Tracer conditions are a less desirable way of achieving control over severity than an index. But the strategy of the drunk who dropped his keys yards away but searches for them under the streetlight seems to apply to tracers: That is where the light is. The most successful research in emergency care to date has used a tracer condition: cardiac arrest. In fact, the study was confined to cases of cardiac arrest due to heart disease occurring out-of-hospital. Using this tracer, it was possible to measure the marginal effectiveness over basic resuscitative care of ALS delivered by paramedics and, in fact, even to determine the importance of time factors, which have a direct and measurable relationship in pre-hospital care to resources required (Eisenberg, Bergner, & Hallstrom, 1980).

The reasons this tracer was so useful illustrate some of the requirements of tracers: It is a fairly frequent condition; it is easy to recognize (the victim falls down, unconscious and pulseless); it is subject to objective confirmation via EKG; it is treatable and has a known and almost certain outcome if untreated; there is a fair amount of agreement on precisely how it should be treated; and, because many episodes are witnessed, it is possible to measure the value of time-to-treatment. It lacks one property that would make it a *true* tracer: The care of this condition is not necessarily representative of emergency care in general or even of all cardiac care. We cannot measure this attribute, a fact which tends to be true of tracers in general and makes them a less-than-perfect tool. It is possible that counterparts to cardiac arrest can be identified among behavioral emergencies; if so, such an approach would provide a beginning. Advances in casefinding tools, such as the SCL-90 (Derogatis et al., 1976) and the "CES-D" depression scale (Radloff, 1977; Weissman, Sholomskas, Pottenger, Prusoff, & Locke, 1977), plus increasing rigor in diagnosing and recording as offered by the "DSM-III" (American Psychiatric Association, 1980), offer some promise that the approach is feasible.

Describing the Care Process

Even if it were not necessary to classify the patient for any other reason, it would have to be done in order to develop an adequate means of measuring or describing the process of care. Structural measures cannot substitute; they bear insufficient relationship either to the care process or to outcome (Brook et al., 1976).

Useful outcome studies cannot be done without accounting for variations in the care process from clinician to clinician, from setting to setting, and over time. Even if this were not the case, simply knowing that patients (even equivalent patients) in one facility do better than patients in another is not particularly helpful unless you know what makes the difference.[3]

Two basic approaches are available for measuring the care process: (1) concurrent or retrospective methods of evaluating care against some standard and (2) prospective methods of guiding care in compliance with some standard. The first approach depends absolutely upon the quality and completeness of data, including patient records; the second, likewise, requires good records in order to be able to detect deviations from the standard, but it also implies a high degree of control over the setting. In either case, the absolute requirement is for an *explicit standard of care*.

Retrospective audit was used to measure the performance of basic-level EMTs (those who have received the standard 81-hour training program) by Frazier and Cannon (1978). The investigators used the training curriculum and materials to devise a standard which consisted of "mandated treatments." A mandated treatment is one which is (1) observable and (2) always required upon identification of a specific condition. For example, a suspected fracture is always to be splinted. Whether or not the mandated treatment is demonstrably related to improved outcome is not the issue; the basic question is, Are the EMTs complying with prescribed treatments? This simple approach has limitations: It relies upon the ambulance trip report, and hence is only as good as the self-report of actions which this record (or any medical record) contains. Furthermore, it does not permit any assessment of whether the splint was put on correctly, whether the correct splint was used, whether it was put on while the patient was expiring due to an obstructed airway, or whether it took two EMTs ten minutes to do a job that should have required three minutes of one EMT's time. Studies using observers with carefully designed instruments are currently underway, which may provide sufficient additional information to justify the expense (Sechrest, 1979).

A more direct method of controlling the care process is to guide the care prospectively. An interesting example in emergency care illustrates several issues that are as relevant to behavioral emergencies as to the surgical emergencies with which the study is directly concerned. The research is being carried out at Yale-New Haven Hospital (Frazier & Brand, 1979). It centers on a series of care algorithms (step-by-step guides to care, employing branching logic). The first algorithm was for soft-tissue lacerations, a very frequent surgical emergency. It was first developed as a tool for auditing the medical record, but it soon became apparent that the medical record was so incomplete that a meaningful audit could not be carried out in the great majority of cases. The standard record was then replaced by a checklist based upon the algorithm. That step alone achieved a dramatic increase in completeness of the record, so that only a small percentage of cases was unauditable.[4] The next step was to bring the care process into compliance with the standard; a randomly assigned study group of physicians received rapid feedback via a computer printout which noted deviations from the algorithm (the algorithm itself was available to both the study and control house staff). Results showed a dramatic effect upon compliance which increased with repeated messages; some of this improvement persisted when the feedback was terminated. Additional algorithms are being developed and tested for four other conditions: burns, soft-tissue infections, and upper- and lower-extremity injuries.

Originally, the major objective of the research was to study the effect upon outcome of care that met the standard versus care that deviated. That objective, as an immediate aim, has been abandoned. Soft-tissue lacerations, at least at Yale, have a readily measurable bad outcome (i.e., infection) in only about three percent of the cases. Other outcomes, such as extent of scarring, are difficult to measure and become apparent only long after the patient has left the scene. On the other hand, serious burns and soft-tissue infections have fairly frequent bad outcomes, but the condition is seen so infrequently as to require years of observation before any significant effect of care will be identifiable.

Another important point is brought out in the process used to develop the standard: where it exists, empirical research and results of controlled clinical trials should provide the basis for the standard. Where it does not, one attempts to create or identify some kind of consensus on the part of clinicians. Where consensus cannot be obtained, provided the question is not trivial (e.g., what color the suturing material should be), a question emerges which represents a high priority for controlled clinical trial. Furthermore, a setting in which algorithms are employed to standardize the care process is excellent for controlled trials of procedures, assuming that outcome data can be collected over an adequate time period to achieve the numbers required (Brand & Frazier, 1979).

In any case, before outcome research can be both feasible and useful, it is generally necessary to be able to measure or control for variation in the care process. This can be done only to the extent that some method exists for classifying the patient in terms of the kind of care needed and urgency of the need. There are, of course, additional requirements for outcome research; a reasonably powerful design to some extent can reduce the requirements for patient and process description.

It also helps to have an extremely powerful intervention. A case in point is the study in King County, Washington (Eisenberg et al., 1980). The combination of cardiopulmonary resuscitation (CPR) and ALS is, evidently, able to achieve very large differences in survival from cardiac arrest, as compared with CPR alone. Also, of course, the study condition is well defined. ALS treatment for cardiac arrest is straight-forward, well recorded in these Seattle suburbs, and carried out according to fairly uniform protocol, although the skill with which it is done may vary widely. CPR is not carried out uniformly or by people with uniform training. It is performed not only by trained and experienced EMTs, but by members of the public who are present when an arrest occurs. Many Seattle residents have had an abbreviated course in CPR, but often it is done with apparent good effect by untrained bystanders who have merely seen it enacted on television or read about it in newspapers. Nevertheless, because of the fairly strong quasi-experimental design it was possible to employ, plus the strength of the treatment and precision of case definition, variations in the skill with which the treatment was carried out could be dismissed as important sources of the differences in outcome. Also, the research is able to address long-term survival (not just survival to emergency department admission) on the questionable assumption that all the hospitals of destination had coronary care units and all coronary care units provide equivalent care; only the exceptional conditions previously mentioned make it possible to rule out variations in inpatient care as sources of variation in survival to hospital discharge or beyond. In effect, this model, applied to care of behavioral emergencies, again argues that the way to begin is with a "good" (that is, frequent and easily recognized) condition with a "good" (both well-defined and powerful) treatment.

Summary

Behavioral emergencies probably represent a large category of need which currently appears to be met very poorly in both the general health and the mental health systems. It is probably a category of demand which places a heavy, perhaps growing, burden upon the emergency medical services system. Depending upon how they are defined, behavioral emergencies may have important consequences, not only to the people who have the behavioral disorders, but to society as a whole.

The above discussion offers a strategy whereby research can contribute ways of improving care of behavioral emergencies. The strategy is keyed to the EMS system, which may be the area in which the general health and the mental health systems are, de facto, most closely linked. The strategy hinges upon measuring the effectiveness of the EMS system, with emphasis upon classifying the patient and describing the care process. These steps are seen as useful in themselves and as necessary before outcome research can or should be attempted. Only if the capability exists to measure effectiveness is there a rational basis for improvements in the care system. Attempts to evaluate or manage systems for "productivity" or "cost-efficiency," lacking measures of effectiveness which systematically address quality of care, are seen as an inevitable—and dangerous—consequence of delay in this area.

Notes

1. Given such a measure, it may then be possible to go beyond effectiveness to estimate impact, which is the effect upon the population as a whole, an important consideration in planning and financing social programs.

2. There are several dozen possible citations here; an example is Gibson, Anderson, & Bugbee, 1970. Gibson (1973) has also been an early and provocative analyst of the possible causes and implications of the use of emergency departments as sources of primary care.

3. This is not to say that monitoring of outcomes is of no value. Brook (1978) discusses use of outcome measures "to watch what happens in your system to see if there are any problems you can correct." He notes that their use in this way reduces design and analytic requirements, as compared with their use in policy analysis, efficacy, or effectiveness studies.

4. There are other ways of dealing with missing data. Greenfield, for example (1978), uses a probabilistic estimate of whether or not a procedure was carried out but not recorded.

References

American Psychiatric Association. *Diagnostic and statistical manual of mental disorders.* Washington, D.C., 1980.

Barry, W. S., Kharabi, F., Nyman, G., & Schmidt, C. W. Expanding psychiatric service in a hospital emergency room. *Journal of the American Medical Association,* 1979, 242, 1394-1395.

Barton, G. American Psychiatric Task Force on Emergency Care Issues. Presented at the National Symposium on Emergency Medical Services, Denver, Colorado, November 13-16, 1979.

Bigelow, D., Brodsky, G., & Hallgren, E. *A management information system for community mental health.* Unpublished manuscript, Oregon State Mental Health Division, 1978.

Boone, Young and Associates. Study to determine appropriate methodology for developing process measures in emergency care. Final report, Contract No. (HRA) 106-74-138, National Center for Health Services Research. Springfield, VA: National Technical Information Service, PB 250 973, 1975.

Brand, D. A., & Frazier, W. H. Impact of computer-assisted audit on physician performance in an emergency service. In A. Alperovitch, F. T. DeDombal, & F. Gremy (Eds.), *Evaluation of efficacy of medical action.* Amsterdam: Elsevier North-Holland, 1979.

Brook, R. H. *Quality of care assessment: A comparison of five methods of peer review.* DHEW Publication No. (HRA) 74-3100. Hyattsville, MD: National Center for Health Services Research, 1973.

Brook, R. H. *The use of outcome data in EMS research.* Emergency medical services research methodology workshop 2. National Center for Health Services Research, Research Proceedings Series. Dulles International Airport, June 7-8. DHEW Publication No. (PHS) 79-3225-2. Hyattsville, Maryland, 1978.

Brook, R. H., Avery, A. D., Greenfield, S., Harris, L. J., Lelah, T., Solomon, N. E., & Ware, J. E. *Quality of medical care assessment using outcome measures: An overview of the method.* Rand Note R-2021-HEW. Santa Monica, CA: Rand Corporation, 1976.

Brook, R. H., Kamberg, C. J., & Lohr, K. N. *Quality assessment in mental health.* Rand Note N-1206-HEW. Santa Monica, CA: Rand Corporation, 1979.

Buck, G., Brimmer, P., & Putzier, L. T. Emergency medical services research: Effectiveness of emergency care. Final report, Contract No. (HRA) 230-75-0214, National Center for Health Services Research. Springfield, VA: National Technical Information Service, PB 262-766, 1976.

Champion, H. R., & Sacco, W. *Triage by protocol.* Emergency medical services research methodology workshop 2. National Center for Health Services Research, Research Proceedings Series. Dulles International Airport, June 7-8. DHEW Publication No. (PHS) 79-3225-2. Hyattsville, Maryland, 1979.

Ciarlo, J., & Reihman, J. *The Denver community mental health questionnaire: Development of a multidimensional program evaluation instrument.* Denver: Northwest Denver Community Mental Health Center, 1974.

Derogatis, L. R., Rickels, K., & Rock, A. F. The SCL-90 and the MMPI: A step in the validation of a new self-report scale. *British Journal of Psychiatry,* 1976, 128, 280-289.

Eisenberg, M. S., Bergner, L., & Halstrom, A. Out-of-hospital cardiac arrest: Improved survival with paramedic services. *Lancet,* 1980, 1, 812-815.

Fauman, B. J. Psychiatry in the emergency "room." *Journal of the American Medical Association,* 1979, 242, 1401.

Frazier, W. H., & Brand, D. A. Quality assessment and the art of medicine: The anatomy of laceration care. *Medical Care,* 1979, 17, 5.

Frazier, W. H., & Cannon, J. F. *Emergency medical technician performance evaluation.* National Center for Health Services Research, Research Report Series. DHEW Publication No. (PHS) 78-3211. Hyattsville, Maryland, 1978.

Gibson, G. The social system of emergency care. In J. Nobel (Ed.), *Emergency medical services: Behavioral and planning perspectives.* New York: Behavioral Publications, 1973.

Gibson, G., Anderson, O. W., & Bugbee, G. *Emergency medical services in the Chicago area.* Chicago: University of Chicago Center for Health Administration Studies, 1970.

Greenfield, S. Assessing emergency systems quality: Method development. In *Emergency medical services systems research projects, 1978.* National Center for Health Services Research, Research Management Series. DHEW Publication No. (PHS) 79-3220. Hyattsville, Maryland, 1978.

Gustafson, D., & Halloway, D. C. A decision theory approach to measuring severity in illness. *Health Services Research,* 1975, 10, 97.

Hall, R. C. W. Psychiatric emergencies and physical illness: A forgotten relationship. Presented at the Twelfth Annual Taylor Manor Hospital Psychiatric Symposium, Ellicott City, Maryland, April 12, 1980.

Jacobs, J. *The emergency services workshop—A summary of proceedings, December 1-2, 1977.* Rockville, MD: National Institute of Mental Health, 1977.

Kiresuk, T., & Sherman, R. Goal attainment scaling: A general method for evaluating community mental health programs. *Community Mental Health Journal,* 1968, 6, 22-41.

Krischer, J. P. Indexes of severity: Underlying concepts. *Health Services Research,* 1976, 11, 143-157.

McKenzie, E., Gibson, G., & Garthe, E. Evaluating the abbreviated injury scale. Presented at the annual meeting of the American Public Health Association, Washington, D.C., 1977.

Newman, F. L., Burwell, B. A., & Underhill, W. E. Program analysis using the client oriented cost outcome system. *Evaluation and Planning Journal,* 1978, 1, 19-30.

Nutt, P. Burn care standards. *Wisconsin Medical Journal,* 1974, 73, 37-42.

Psychiatric News. New CMHC survey shows better emergency service. August 19, 1977, p. 16.

Radloff, L. S. The CES-D scale: A self-report depression scale for research in the general population. *Applied Psychological Measurement,* 1977, 1, 385-401.

Schainblatt, A. H. *Monitoring the outcomes of state mental health treatment programs: Some initial suggestions.* Washington, DC: The Urban Institute, 1977.

Sechrest, L. B. Measurement of EMT performance. In *Emergency medical services systems research projects, 1978*. National Center for Health Services Research, Research Management Series. DHEW Publication No. (PHS) 79-3220. Hyattsville, Maryland, 1979.

Weissman, M. M., Sholomskas, D., Pottenger, M., Prusoff, B., & Locke, B. F. Assessing depressive symptoms in five psychiatric populations: A validation study. *American Journal of Epidemiology,* 1977, 106, 203-214.

About the Contributors

C. Clifford Attkisson is Associate Professor of Psychology at the University of California, San Francisco. He earned his A.B. degree at the University of Richmond and in 1970 was awarded the Ph.D. degree in psychology by the University of Tennessee. His graduate work focused on clinical and community psychology. During the past nine years his teaching, research, and publications have concentrated on the areas of program evaluation, information systems for the human services, and psychotherapy research. Currently he is a core faculty member in the Health Psychology graduate program at UCSF and is director of the Program Evaluation Service of the District V Mental Health Center in San Francisco. Dr. Attkisson is coeditor of *Resource Materials for Community Mental Health Program Evaluation* (1977) and senior editor of *Evaluation of Human Service Programs* published in 1978 by Academic Press. He also is an associate editor of the *Journal of Health Psychology*.

Jerry Authier is a practicing psychotherapist and Associate Professor of Medical Psychology in the Departments of Family Practice and Psychiatry at the University of Nebraska Medical Center in Omaha. He received his Ph.D. in psychology from the University of Portland, Oregon in 1973. His professional interests include characteristics differentiating the effective from the ineffective therapist, the microcounseling paradigm, and psychoeducation. He is the author of several articles in this field, and is co-author of the second edition of *Microcounseling, Innovations in Interviewing, Counseling, Psychotherapy and Psychoeducation*.

Anthony Broskowski received his Ph.D. in clinical psychology in 1967 from Indiana University. He has served on the faculty of the University of Pittsburgh and the Harvard Medical School, Laboratory of Community Psychiatry. He is currently Executive Director of the Northside Community Mental Health Center in Tampa, Florida and Associate Professor at the University of South Florida, College of Medicine. He has published extensively in the areas of community psychiatry, program evaluation, and management, including a recent text entitled *Information*

Systems for Health and Human Services coauthored by Cliff Attkisson. He recently served as prime contractor for the NIMH evaluation of the Primary Health Care Project-Community Mental Health Center Initiative. He has served as a consultant to numerous state and federal government agencies and other nonprofit service organizations, and teaches courses on management and evaluation for the NIMH Staff College.

Simon H. Budman is a staff psychologist at the Harvard Community Health Plan in Boston, Massachusetts, where he also directs the Mental Health Research Program. In addition, Dr. Budman is on the faculty of the Harvard Medical School. After receiving his doctorate in clinical psychology from the University of Pittsburgh, he was on the faculty of the University of Rochester Medical School and then the Boston University Medical School. He is the guest editor (with Donald Wertlieb) of a special issue of *Professional Psychology* on "Psychologists in Health Care Settings," and himself edited *Forms of Brief Therapy* (New York: Guilford Press, 1981). Dr. Budman has published numerous articles and book chapters on health psychology, psychotherapy research, group psychotherapy, and brief treatment.

Jack D. Burke, Jr., is Research Psychiatrist in the Primary Care Research Section of NIMH, where he has worked on projects examining the BCHS-NIMH Linkage Initiative and the clinical practice of primary care clinicians. He received his B.A., M.D., and M.P.H. degrees from Harvard University and trained in psychiatry at Massachusetts Mental Health Center and in social psychiatry at Massachusetts General Hospital.

Barbara J. Burns is Chief of the Primary Care Research Section at the National Institute of Mental Health. She also holds appointments as Consultant in Psychology in the Department of Psychiatry, Massachusetts General Hospital, and as Instructor of Psychology, Harvard Medical School. Previously she directed the mental health services of the Bunker Hill Health Center of the MGH, a neighborhood health center, where she also conducted studies on the provision of mental health services in the context of general health care. She has also been a director of child mental health services at the Erich Lindemann Mental Health Center in Boston, Massachusetts, and has taught graduate students at Boston College and the Harvard School of Public Health.

Nancy Marwick DeMuth is a postdoctoral research fellow at Johns Hopkins University 1980-81, and is on leave from her position as Assistant Professor of Management and Health Care at Pennsylvania State University. She received her Ph.D. in counseling psychology from the University of Utah and a M.B.A. from the Wharton School at the University of Pennsylvania. Current research interests are in the areas of professional stress management, economics and psychotherapy, cost-effectiveness analysis of mental health systems, and behavioral correlates of hypertension. Dr. DeMuth's work in economics and psychotherapy has resulted in two recent articles, one coauthored with Edna Kamis in the *Journal of Consulting and Clinical Psychology* and the other coauthored with Brian T. Yates in *Professional Psychology*. She has taught courses primarily in the areas of organizational behavior, health care delivery systems, and mental health evaluation and planning. Dr. De-Muth is also a practicing family and individual psychotherapist and does consulting with physicians and dentists in the areas of practice management.

Robert P. Ehrlich is currently a psychology intern at Northside Community Mental Health Center in Tampa, Florida. He received his M.S. and Ph.D. in human development and family studies from the Pennsylvania State University. Dr. Ehrlich has coauthored several articles and papers relating to The Community Helpers Project, a project designed to assess the help-giving and help-seeking behavior of rural residents and to establish a community-based program to enhance natural helping networks. His current activities include training mental health personnel to work in primary health care settings, developing and evaluating a mass media campaign focused on prevention and the promotion of health, and enhancing the informal support networks of deinstitutionalized psychiatric patients.

Gene V Glass is Professor of Education at the University of Colorado-Boulder. He received his doctorate in educational psychology from the University of Wisconsin in 1965. He is a past president of the American Educational Research Association. His research interests involve social science methodology, statistics, evaluation research, and the relationship between psychotherapy and medical utilization. He authored *Design and Analysis of Time-Series Experiments* (with V. L. Willson and J. M. Gottman), *Benefits of Psychotherapy* (with M. L. Smith and T. I. Miller), and *Overtreated and Underserved: The High Cost of Medical Priorities* (with H. J. Schlesinger and E. Mumford). He is editor of the first volume of the *Sage Evaluation Studies Review Annual*.

Eric N. Goplerud is presently Manager of Program Planning and Evaluation at Northside Community Mental Health Center in Tampa, Florida. He holds a Ph.D. in clinical/community psychology from the State University of New York at Buffalo. He has interests in the development of self-help groups and natural support networks as mediators of life stress, the establishment of community-based alternatives to psychiatric hospitalization for emotionally disturbed persons, and the development and administration of comprehensive health/mental health programs. His previous publications are in the areas of differential diagnosis of functional psychoses, risk for affective psychoses, the negative impact of deinstitutionalization, effects of stress and social support systems, and cross-cultural patterns of mental health organization.

Homer J. Hagedorn is Manager of Organization Development at Arthur D. Little, Inc., in Cambridge, Massachusetts. He has directed numerous program evaluation projects for NIMH and the Health Resources Administration (DHHS), as well as planning studies and other consultative assignments at federal, state, and local levels. His Ph.D. was awarded in American history by Harvard University in 1955. His dissertation described the life and times of a management consultant. His recent publications include two manuals published by NIMH: *A Working Manual of Simple Program Evaluation Techniques for Community Mental Health Centers* (1976) and *A Manual on State Mental Health Planning* (1977).

Linda Heard Hollen is Program Manager of the Outpatient Department at Northside Community Mental Health Center in Tampa, Florida and Clinical Instructor of Psychiatry at the University of South Florida College of Medicine. She received an M.Ed. in counseling from American University. Ms. Hollen's research interests include family therapy and health-mental health linkages. She is Codirector of the Community Mental Health for Family Physicians training project.

Larry G. Kessler is currently a statistician in the Primary Care Research Section of the Applied Biometrics Research Branch, Division of Biometry and Epidemiology, NIMH. He received his B.S. degree in mathematics from Boston University and his D.S. degree in operations research from the Johns Hopkins University, School of Hygiene and Public Health. Subsequent to receiving his doctorate, he was employed as a health research scientist at the Veterans Administration Health Services Research and Development Center, Perry Point, Maryland. He is also an associate in the Division of Operations Research, Department of Health Services Administration, School of Hygiene and Public Health, the Johns Hopkins University.

James S.J. Manuso holds a Ph.D. in psychology from the Graduate School of Political and Social Science of the New School for Social Research. He is Director of The Equitable Life Assurance Society's New York-based Emotional Health Program and founder of industry's first in-house Biofeedback Laboratory. He is internationally recognized for his work in corporate emotional health programs and policies and in the recognition, prevention, treatment, and costs of corporate stress overloads. He has taught, written, and spoken extensively in these fields, having served as an advisor to the President's Commission on Mental Health and to the Senate Subcommittee on Health and Scientific Research. He recently completed the book, *Stress Management Training in a Large Corporation*, and the film, "Managing Stress."

Edward Marks is a doctoral candidate in clinical community psychology at the University of South Florida, where he also received his M.A. degree. He received his B.A. in psychology at Washington University, St. Louis. His research interests include the relationship between psychological status and health, the development of interorganizational relationships for the delivery of health and mental health care, and the evaluation of mental health programs. He coordinated the preliminary evaluation of the federal government's Primary Health Care Project-Community Mental Health Center Linkage Initiative, and has conducted a number of program evaluations within community mental health settings.

Emily Mumford is Professor of Psychiatry and Preventive Medicine at the University of Colorado School of Medicine. She received her M.A. and Ph.D. in sociology from Columbia University. She is the principal investigator on an NIMH project to develop methods of analyzing the ability of student physicians to recognize psychological and social problems of general medical patients and deal with them effectively in brief encounters. Her published works include *Interns: From Student to Physician, Sociology in Hospital Care,* a forthcoming book, *Social Science Perspectives in Health and Illness,* and numerous papers on psychological and social factors in medical education and in the delivery of health services. With Gene Glass and Herbert Schlesinger, she coauthored a series of papers and a forthcoming book, *Overtreated and Underserved,* on the subject of cost-offset of mental health treatments.

Herbert J. Schlesinger is Professor of Psychiatry at the University of Colorado School of Medicine, Chief of the Psychology Service at the Denver Veterans Administration and Medical Center, and Training and Supervising Analyst at the Denver Institute for Psychoanalysis. He is also Editor of *Psychological Issues Monograph Series.* He received his Ph.D. from the University of Kansas and for many years was at the Menninger Foundation. His recent research has been on the effects of mental health treatment on utilization of medical care services, in which he has been associated with Emily Mumford, Gene V Glass, and Cathleen Patrick.

George C. Stone is Professor of Medical Psychology at the University of California, San Francisco and Director of the Graduate Academic Program in Psychology there. He received his Ph.D. in experimental/physiological psychology from the University of California, Berkeley, and after brief periods at the University of Illinois and at the G. D. Searle company in Skokie, Illinois, where he established a psychopharmacology laboratory, he moved to the Langley Porter Psychiatric Institute and the University of California, San Francisco. His interests encompass the area of learning-cognition-communication, and he has approached these topics with techniques ranging from the physiological to the social. He has participated actively in the development of the new field of health psychology, and is senior author of the book *Health Psychology* and editor of a new journal, also called *Health Psychology,* that will begin publication in 1982 under the auspices of Division 38 (Health Psychology) of the American Psychology Association.

Elinor Walker is Health Scientist Administrator in the National Center for Health Service Research, Office of Health Research, Statistics and Technology, Department of Health and Human Services. She has a B.A. from the University of Maryland and studied at the University of North Carolina School of Public Health. Ms. Walker is engaged in the extramural research program of NCHSR in emergency medical services, and is particularly interested in developing a research in effectiveness of care of behavioral emergencies.

Donald Wertlieb, Ph.D., is a clinical developmental psychologist on the staff of the Judge Baker Guidance Center, Harvard Medical School. He is Assistant Professor in the Eliot-Pearson Department of Child Study, Tufts University, and Senior Research Associate at the Harvard Community Health Plan. Among his interests are the impact of life stress upon family health care utilization and development of interventions designed to alleviate such stress.

Stephen L. White is Executive Director of the Pawtucket-Central Falls Community Mental Health Center in Pawtucket, Rhode Island. He was formerly Deputy Director at Northside Community Mental Health Center in Tampa, Florida and Clinical Assistant Professor of Psychiatry at the University of South Florida College of Medicine. He holds an M.S.W. from Smith College for social work and an M.P.A. in health services management from Golden Gate University. Mr. White has published widely in the areas of family therapy, mental health policy, and human services management. He is the editor of *Middle Management in Mental Health* (Jossey-Bass, 1980) and the author of *Managing Health and Human Services Programs* (Free Press, 1981).

Brian T. Yates received his Ph.D. in psychology from Stanford University in 1976 and his B.A. in psychology from the University of California at San Diego. He has published or has in press 21 articles in basic, applied, evaluation, and operations research. Dr. Yates also is the author of *Improving Effectiveness and Reducing Costs in Mental Health* (Charles C Thomas, 1980). He is now writing two more books: a guide to doing the dissertation in psychology, and a practical guide to cost-effectiveness analysis coauthored by Dr. Fred Newman. Dr. Yates was the contractor for a recent report on the Cost-Effectiveness of Psychotherapy published in 1980 by the U.S. Congress's Office of Technology Assessment. Assistant Professor of Clinical/Experimental Psychology at the American University in Washington, D.C., he is Director of the Self Management Institute specializing in applying cost-effectiveness analysis and operations research at a personal level to improving community residents' weight, insomnia, and time management.